2015©

As this book reflects a personal observation, of past activities and events, copying for educational studies and/or improvements within the medical facilities, which provide treatment to patients, I must permit readers to use this as a referential guide. Please do not attempt to develop this book furthering your personal aspects; however, sharing in conversation as well as critical thinking, as in a think tank atmosphere, could not destroy my recollections.

Contact: **Lana T. Reddock**, M. of Ed

{*Formerly*: **CEO of Hooked On Yarn, Inc.**}

7314 NW 75th Street

Tamarac FL 33321

1-954-324-9896 (magicJack)

1-954-383-4072 (cell)

First Edition {Printed February 1999}

First Revision {March-April 2003}

Print for Copyright Version {September 2004}

Self-Publishing 2015

Concern for others, study, work, and my experiences comprised this book, along with hours of data processing personal recollections and observations. My advice:

"Stay healthy, this book is a good reason!"

This non-fiction book is a reality for patients: young, aged, disabled, and healthy individuals as well. (I ponder) *"Why do patients have to be treated as if they are last week's trash?"* And, honestly, you should be aware:

"Funding *just another word for money."*

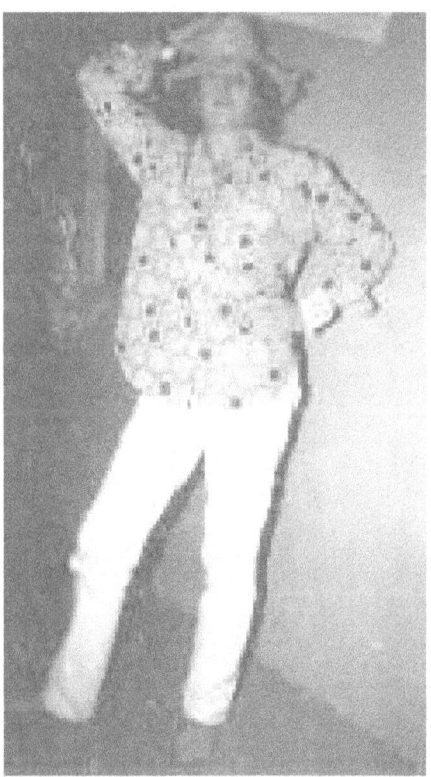

1990 Lana Reddock

Truthfully, do not get sick unless you have connections with GOD!

Table of Contents

Day one of research:

Jessica, a High School sophomore donated 4 hours of her time, to assist in computer research, for the section - Abuse/Treatments

Librarians, Coral Springs FL, they impressed me.; a volunteer was courteous and helpful, asking to assist with our searches. Much to my surprise the volunteer, as Jessica and I were leaving, mentioned we impressed the staff as well, by our ability to seek and find data on our own, most of the time. Actually, we merely were pulling whimsically, articles in ProQuest. Compliments like that are always encouraging.

Honestly, all Broward County Librarians, in Tamarac, Fort Lauderdale, Sunrise, and online public library services contributed time, during stressful, research, difficult to access. They are great people; their skills enhanced mine, making improved writing about an extremely sensitive medical care aspect, for not only seniors but any patient requiring care and treatment, or just understanding by a medical professional.

Productive Schedule

prior to July 2015

(that had begun and completed this book)

- Thursday August 27, 1998 Start Time 09:36:12 [Outline Preparation]

- November 1, 1998, this book was finally complete; for future reference.

- It needed only to be proofread and edited.

- Today, Sunday, March 30, 2003 I am revising and editing the book's context, for transmission to a publisher. It is anticipated the editing process will not be longer than one week.

- April 09, 2003 this book is completed; changes, corrections, and updates have been added.

- July 24, 2015 began its self-publishing aspect, to submit for actual printing, after revisions.

- August 27th 2015 created a glossary, to define specific related terms

- September 27th 2015 finally 'proofreading and editing phase'

Introduction

My name is on the cover {but} it is not who I am? Truthfully, I am the innovator, researcher, observer, and author of this book; several other books are considered by me to be: <u>collectives</u>.

There were times while writing, I wanted to use a fictitious name; I just could not think of a suitable one. Knowledge is something I have increased with age because of as noted earlier; a childhood injury brought many closed doors my way. The injury began a lifetime desire to record only a few of the horrible experiences. Sharing my past was not to become part of this book; therefore, to focus upon remembered events <u>as a patient</u> back then may seem arrogant currently. During the 1950s and most recently, in the 21st century similarities in professional negativity, for myself as well as others makes for interesting reading.

The events, negative and positive were at times horrifying. This book, along with the internet and periodical media filled with articles can continue to advance knowledge. Self-skills and preventive unnecessary care, at continual rising-costs have become doom throughout lifetimes. The 1990's patients differ from previous decades; all of which seemed to surface and to self-improve, upon the public's awareness, for short times.

Elderly today have changed from being afraid to come out of their homes, into new men and women. Not only Americans are becoming brave and standing on their own two feet; there are men and women of International and Global Cultures awakening, to the needs of their loved-ones and themselves.

Disabled (previously identified as *handicapped*) - once thought of as less than capable are given legal opportunities, to defend their rights. Malpractice injuries through negligence of parental incompetence, medical errors, and related reasons have predominantly infuriated medical facility professionals; therefore, changes have surfaced with reassessments and reevaluations – to provide insight to decrease mismanagement, related to improper care, diagnosis, and treatment. Mentally Deficient has replaced the disable, for the uneducated individual requiring constant leadership. Deaf, mute, blind, and amputees have surfaced into a new century (in this 21st century) – to find much more available and adaptable services within local neighborhoods.

Patients requiring a medical facility/private care center have learned to seek qualified professionals; administrators, scientists, diagnosticians, physicians, nurses, housekeepers and dieticians of every level, not merely professionally. Today, that is more visible than ever, regarding the use of preventive-illnesses; the patient of minimal, maximum, or an ordinary office visit – as a preventive finds requiring healthcare and medicine both have rising costs. Many insurance companies limit the quantitative supplies monthly; however, co-payments have increased available prescription medications, to patients on fixed-income (i.e.: retirees, young adult parents and single parent household, and of course emergency victims). It appears healthiness is alive-and-well only to those with insurance, savings, and assets that they are willing to pay, for a fairly good future. And in 2015, President Obama made available a nationwide insurance coverage, designed to meet the needs of individuals on less than a high-salaried income. This plan had its setbacks early on; therefore, only a small percentage of Americans have been qualified, to be covered. The improvements to the internet accessible service, since the major website problems has improved, opening venues less stressfully and providing a scaled-monthly contribution – for eligible households.

Patients in **wheelchairs** are encouraged to participate, in activities for both their mental and physical health, to maintain social and local activities. Sports are becoming prominent factors, in developing better-and-less conspicuous prosthetic devices, for amputees. There is a realistic over-all-view connecting health and daily care, by laypersons and professionals. The world is becoming a better place, to live for the once thought-of as: old, sickly, handicapped, mentally debilitated, and others.

Adolescents becoming independent often of their parents and guardians are selecting managers and agents, as promotional entrepreneurs, in their diverse aspects of technologies and creative inventions. A multitude of modern adolescents - those of the

1980s, 1990s and continuing into this 21st Century - know ways to get help; other than 911 during a major crisis. They are not afraid to pick and choose friends.

Some select new parental figures; divorcing legally or inconspicuously their natural or guardians. Many have good reasons. Others have small concerns - out of the normally anticipated minor quirks - impossible they believe can be dealt with by educators or other professional personnel. And perhaps there may continue to be students fed up at a young age, they never will find their niche'.

The old saying: "*Go to your room*," has reversed; it backfired, on many parents; perhaps, for the better. A difference of opinion on topics about the *'kids'* place, *'grownups'* place, healthy or sick place created any intensity for living, at home and within numerous neighborhoods. The result led the way to understanding individuals and patients require a hug, communication, or to be among others with similar fears, doubts and sorrows, reinvented community-style living. It is a creative way to help others and we, as a team, live together harmoniously. As a patient during the 1950s, I observed unprofessional treatment to others, and myself, in a hospital.

The purpose of writing this book was to compare way back when care to the present time; to clear the cobwebs in my mind of clutter, filling me with fear - for the safety of myself and others - would have been a personal plus. This book began as a personal-study of changes, improvements, and outlooks, for future patients, requiring temporary care and treatment. Long-term residents not sickly, just aged, in assisted as well as residential medical facilities might be able to enjoy the aging process, but as I have found thus far that dream of mine is farfetched.

Instead comparisons of my five decades as a long-term scarred patient, my research and memories retain a half a century long gone, which has contributed primarily to a high price, for happiness. A price that cannot be assessed in any monetary aspect; having physical scars that are attached with psychological aches and pains makes life's tomorrow almost as restless as the years passed.

During employment

- Unable to complain formally {*because*} I was not respected; *because* I was too young to have been perceived as knowledgeable - many things I found horrendous and in-humane were not discussed, nor deterred, by the pyramidal staff in a few positions, in medical facilities where I also found the administrative personnel was more interested in their financial income.

- Administrative individuals had minimal if any care or concern, for their patients. Having no one to convey the misery patients endured became a personal nagging thought, especially when someone I knew had to go to a hospital, for a test or diagnostic procedure. I remember being insulted by upper management when I was nineteen or so; I applied for a job, included the following requested crap:
  "I was a parent with children, no diploma, but personal lifetime experience, in and around sick people, for more than a decade. The interviewer damn near laughed at me. I did convince the person to employ me because I was anticipating returning to a school, for nursing within the year."

Such insults to young adults in need of wanted to contribute and to receive respect, finds itself in the shadows of doom. Knowing the difference between 'good care' and 'neglectful treatments' was supposed to be the most important part, of nursing aide's work. For nurses, doctors, and technicians, it too was believed to be *their* obligation to their patients. For me, students learning treatments and professional aspects required of medical personnel, it was time-consuming' although it also cost facilities for the training time required, by its staff, to inform and instruct new employees with proper techniques – more often than not in-house training becomes stagnant.

I might as well include more often than I would like to admit I found realistically speaking, for the cost of medical care, *'nobody gives a shit,'* about patients. But, as this century came to its finale' - history mattered little. Its jut that - **history**!

Facility Types

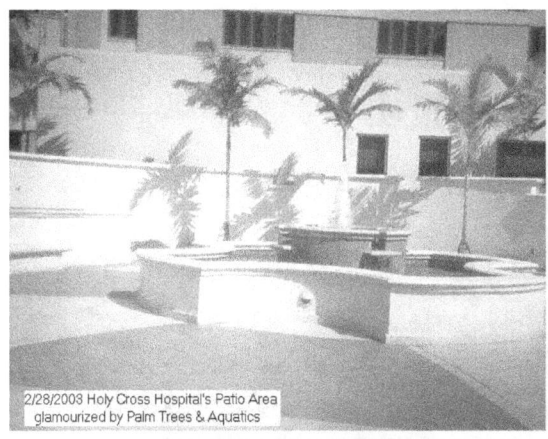

2/28/2003 Holy Cross Hospital's Patio Area glamourized by Palm Trees & Aquatics

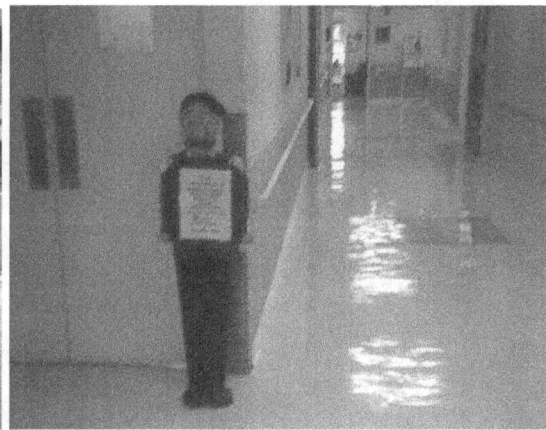

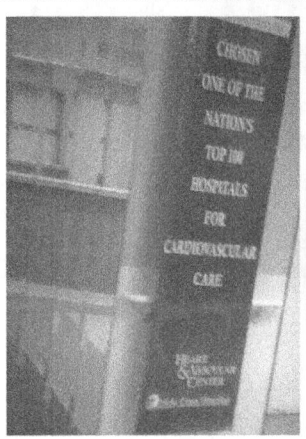

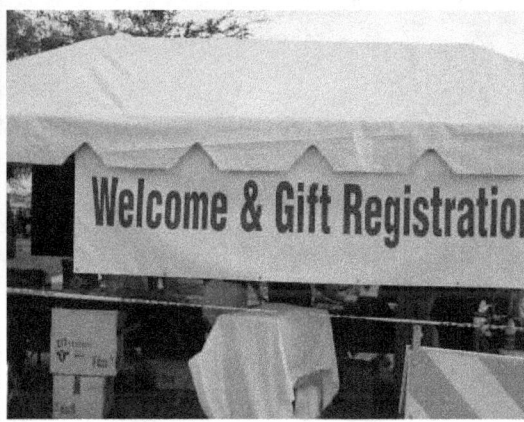

2003 Holy Cross Hospital, Ft Lauderdale FL

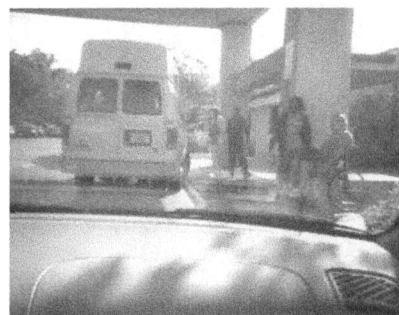

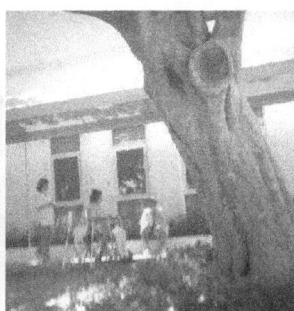

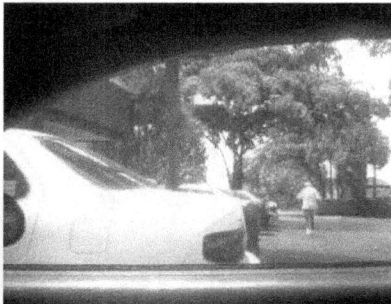

2003 Sunrise FL Convalescent Home

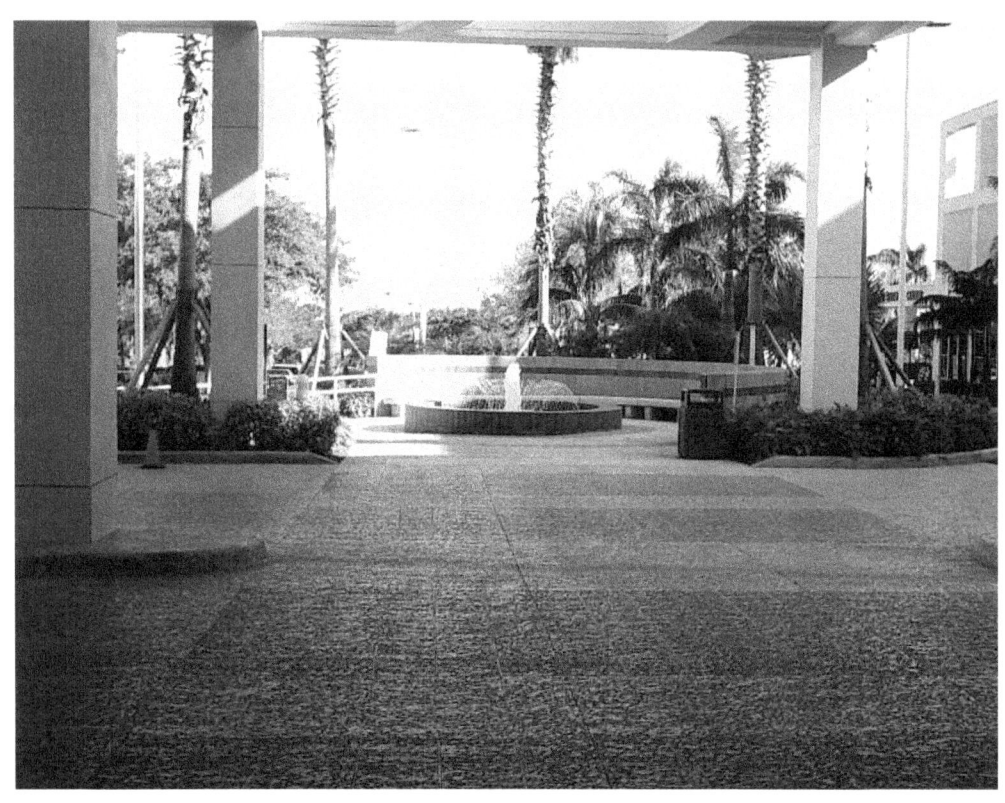

2006 University Hospital Medical Center Tamarac FL

Just a few images of 'medical facilities' providing patient care and record keeping

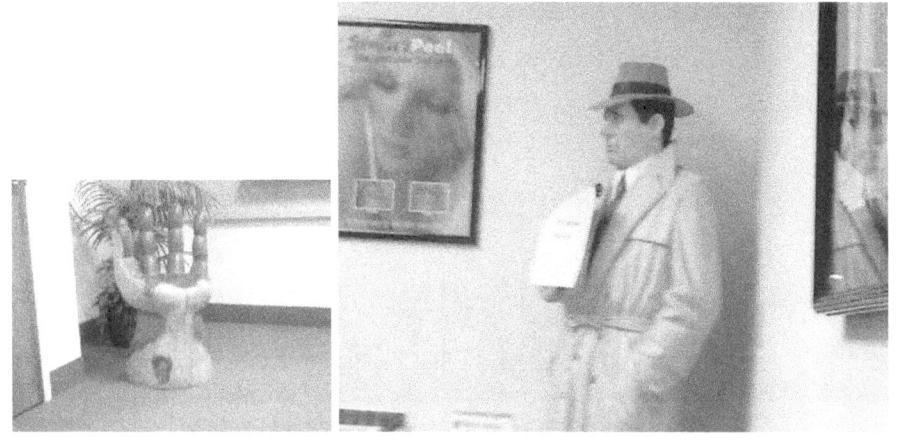

2006 Dermatologist's Patient Waiting Room

Public Treatment Facility A place financed with tax dollars, by community residents usually as an attached assessment cost, for homeowners. Some public or community facilities receive donations, to fund impoverished areas; many submit statistic and other findings to journals, periodicals, newspapers and other medical facilities. Submitted findings data, created for new research and informative textbooks. Educational Centers and schools encourage responsibility for others "at what cost to patients?"

Private Treatment Facilities These places also submit data about patients, for a price to similar channels through public data banks. The reason for admitting a patient to such places, is privacy. My question: "would disease, illness, abuse, or accidental ailments have meaningful guide-lines without restrictions, by regulations?" More to the point, "who dictates the rules or appropriate time to hide facts when malpractice occurs?"

I have found it is the one aspect of action nobody wanted responsibility for, declaring a wrongful action by a nursing or physician care person. Other facility or private personnel also sheltered one another when improper or neglect care occurred. A person or a group to declare mistreatment of patients gets to find a new job because nobody likes a snitch or a whistle blower. When will the rule and regulation creators and maintainers develop that honesty level, preached in religious centers, during youth to its followers within community congregations - and in universities, in non-secular worship places?

The list of' where to get treatment' places / facilities is not absolute; even definitions from a many dictionaries and research guide books inform readers of relatively important words, applied or utilized within numerous scientific-realms. There are clinics, convalescent homes, hospices, hospitals, house, nursing homes, patient care centers, rehabilitation centers, and more than I believe is necessary to include; the dictionary I use describes the following, offering a start for individualized personal research...before, a time of need arises.

- **Clinic** a place as in connection with a medical school or hospital, for treatment of nonresident patients (etc.)

- **Convalescent** home a place to convalesce; to progress toward recovery of health after illness; to grow fully strong

- **Hospice** a facility shelter, often in medical facilities, to permit natural but monitored death

- **Hospital** an institution where injured persons are given medical or surgical treatment (etc.)

- **Nursing home** a private residence or the like equipped to care for the aged or infirmed

- **Private dwelling/residence** a building or place of shelter to live in; a residence {known as: Home Sweet Home when I was a kid}, not anymore

- **Patient** a person who is under medical or surgical treatment and/or care

- **Rehabilitation center** a place to restore to condition of good health, ability to work, or the like.

There are many definitions of words used in the medical field. Seriously, a book would not be large enough to describe every word relating to facility, treatment, symptoms, patient diagnosis, prognosis, and other relative in caring for the ill. In some countries, there are no facilities, to treat the injured; often, the ill is left to die alone. In some areas a neighbor is the healthcare person; minimal knowledge and skills prevail within a concerned but non-skilled worker, at times, increasing damage, rather than promoting the healing process.

Who would have thought-of a house as anything more than a dwelling place; someplace to live, cook, bathe, sleep, invite guests, and maybe relax with a book or family entertainments? A house is frequently considered the place to store and utilize personal belongings, such as: clothing, food, beds, toilet, and things - too big or bulky to be carried in a backpack or truck of a vehicle. According to the dictionary, a house is much more. 'It is a place to live, work, and even more than that.' A person would have to be a scholarly linguist to speak, read, or write 100% correctly, and then, a new book of definitions would create another set of revised descriptions, of popular words and phrases familiar to the average individual. How dumb (my beliefs and statements may seem); but the reality I have found through research of all studies, related to living, dying, and mostly to overcoming successfully, an ailment or persecution, that often attracts insulting, arrogant, and manipulating to the injured.

Various facilities giving treatment to the injured are affiliated with universities, in big cities. Besides studying geriatric health-care, I wanted to study psychology. It was costly and time-consuming, back then in the 1960s and 1970s; I did not wish to incur student loans to finance, what may have become a waste of time and money. My energy and endurance was not high when I evaluated my outlook, for my future. It would have meant dedication; studying long hour's body parts of animals, for practice. Studying test tubes filled with body excretions: *blood, urine, mucous, phlegm, feces*, and whatever. **Additional criteria** was tacked-on: identifying blood vessels, body systems, nerves, muscles & bones, and the organs' utilization, in conjunction to the action and reaction, to flexing as well as purifying blood. Eventually the gory stuff was studied but it was not as impressive, as I had anticipated; the mind's thinking pattern was my concern. I wanted to research growth and development patterns of both genders; comparing changes within the advancements of the aging-process, by years-to-decades. That type of critical concern was frowned upon, not by me. It was brushed over as being incorporative as a trouble-making scheme. Anyone reading this gets the idea.

Words are related 'to what we assume' to be fact. Truthfully, professional words mean nothing to a patient. Physician and staff hold the patients' life in their hands; not your relatives, friends, nor others change the outcome, no matter how many pray or efforts to treat the patient, by the staff themselves. Scary, isn't it? Think it's frightening, guess what? The psychologically impaired can expect even less. They receive sedation 'to relax their mind. Maybe they are thinking: *"I gotta get out-of here."*

The reasons are many and vary, for such occurrences, of the ill effects. Just as the purpose of confinements vary, treatments vary as well. Prognosis depends on test-results, usually in typed written-reports, from technicians in laboratories, staff radiologists, and the centers with *MRI* and *CT* scanning equipment.

Data collected written/verbal information regarding patients or anything revealing something of importance, to somebody. Charting escalates probabilities creating a medical emergency or situation requiring medical care. So how long does this progressively intuitive theoretical pinpointing moment take!?! Anywhere between a few minutes to many hours or even several days.

Analysis primarily begins with your name on the entrance form. Things you say, the way you behave or appear to others, and comments or references by EMTs play the major role, in your dilemma. Vital signs are diagnostic tools, you know: temperature, pulse, blood pressure, and respirations; these convey the status of you physical being at the time you were first located as an injured person. From that moment onwards, you are considered a patient when under a medical teams' care and monitoring occurs at annoying intervals, for diagnostic readings. Visible observations by trained medical workers may hinder or assist you in receiving proper care. Diagnosis is based also on your weight, height, reason for being at the medical facility, and what your physician (if you have one) suggests. Does this create a picture in your mind? Perhaps you will become a statistic when you get sick? Yes, that's about the size of it!

Being psychologically injured can be by an assortment of reason, some may have their mind destroyed by a miserable life. Jealousy, has taken hold of people, causing emotional turmoil. Neighbors on a different level provide hideous complaints which often destroys lives; at times, wrongfully. Others may be unconscious from a fall or head injury; and the most statistically recorded I believe of any reason for hospitalization, is that nasty injury created by automobile accidents. There are of course cardiac arrests, respiratory failures, and fractured bones or muscle spasms but, automobile vehicles create the highest risk factor because there are so many individuals driving.

No matter what the reason, psychology portrays a major-role, in the care and treatment of not only mindful matters; it sets precedence for those being treated, in just about any ailment. A good suggestion, to anyone reading this book: *'if you think you are being coerced into treatment, get real help."*

In various mind-blowing expensive to produce movies, more than 60% of earnings to meet the overhead costs, inform the public viewers of realities they wish not to see. An impact has been pumped into the eyes and ears of viewers through films and documentaries, of the dangers to confinement. For instance: "*One Flew Over the Cuckoo's Nest, HELLO-HELLO, COMA, Nightmare on Elm Street, High Anxiety, On Golden Pond,*" and more delighted audiences throughout the world. My favorite movie is about a tenement neglected, tenants left to fend for themselves; a rotten property owner and some out of space robots fill the screen with sadness, silliness, and satisfaction. Fantasized-views by brilliant individuals interested, in real-world problems. The tenants were rescued not by individuals but by Johnny something or other, a robot and its robot babies. Can you imagine? Who would have believed someone could write such and have it be a successful production? It brought laughter and tears to the viewers.

Take a quick reality check, human beings usually wed (when the time is right), bring babies into the world; some practically refuse to allow them to leave the nest after they're grown, married, and capable of reproducing. I believe I am one of those clingers. It is a gripe all adolescents seem to have but rarely speak to their parents about. Parents do however 'inform their children' but rarely educate them, about safety concerns with any great stabilizing ability. Parents permit public or private schools to do the job. "*But ... why?"* It appears only to complain about the way adolescents act, behave, study, relax, eat, believe, and the list goes on and on, for pages and pages. Let's compare individuals to other things we observe.

Animals survive by finding or killing food, for nourishment; leave the off-spring after a few months or within the first year. How much education can an animal give about surviving? Shelter required by animals is minimal. Animals are vegetarians, primarily; if very hungry, animals will kill small or less aggressive animals, for food. Animals do not cook or season food. People, we season and preserve. Something's got to wrong with human logic, in some respects to their instinctual-survival skills. Animals die when injured if a wound doesn't heal with the procedures used in the jungle. It seems animals are intelligent.

Plants have no shelter for big trees that cover small ones, shrubs and vegetation if planted correctly. Gardens get shelter when owners apply synthetic products and good landscaping techniques. Individuals fertilize vegetables to enlarge growth. Fruit trees get fertilized with insecticides [along with other garden plants] to prevent and reduce diseases, from flying or crawling insects. *"But, what about poison?"* Most individuals do when serving others or feeding a child, to set a good stand, wash or wipe away the surface before it can be eaten.

Human beings are probably filled with pesticides, but it does not seem to matter much. How funny, how stupid and weird; but very much so true! This book is just a long, dragged out opinion of truths and personal thoughts. The comparison of humans, animals, and plants is getting scary.

Care half-heartedly and neglectful observations has me baffled because it too is scary; more than real comparisons of life in any lower or higher life form.

The research along with personal observations made this book, individuals worthy. I have found many individuals do not think about their future until they are in their late forties or early fifties... Next week, for some is far away. As a young spouse (till the relationship ended) I was a parent as my life filled with concern for my family, relatives, and friends. Thoughts of some time in the future was predominant, with questions of:

1.   *Where would I be in twenty years?*

2.   *What about the effect of my life; how would my working help or destroy - my kids' youthfulness?*

3.   *Would they lack good parental guidance?*

4.   *How could they nicely be told - 'the world was a bitterly and distraught place' - for all people, young and old?*

5. *How could the adolescents and zillions of others be informed of the crude things, occurring to decent and innocent individuals?"*

I didn't have the guts when they were very young to say, "*Nobody gives a shit about us;*" or "*strangers only want money for groceries, clothing, taxable, non-taxables, medical treatment, prescriptions, over the counter stuff, and all the other things we too spent money on.*"

After a bickering moment in particular, those words blurted out. Yep, all about "*how rotten the world was for me, a more or less stranded mother.*" Must have scared them half to death, but there's only so much a person under pressure can do to balance work, family, and any kind of personal sanity for personal growth. Minutes of shouting, ranting, and raving for what must have seemed an eternity has also been said, by many other parents. It was not proper to just say whatever I thought (back then or whenever). Kids' demands and expectations of their parents, of their educators, and friends, is quite high; they want rewards, no matter how simple desired, rarely insight of the difficulties surrounding them. Parents are supposed to be calm, caring, understanding, and all that. Perhaps the idiom: *"...been there, seen it, and done that but don't remember,"* explains many people's point of views. It may be a self-defense mechanism.

It was true many nursing assistants and aides hated their jobs. Individuals working with the elderly, handicapped, or long-term terminal patients were a special-breed. They had more than a strong back and weak mind; they needed to be rewarded with an extra hour for lunch; an additional day off and more. Aides didn't have to be told it's time to do a task. The obligation or responsibility came with the daily-knowledge of awareness, individuals in a facility worked! Supervisors disclosed their thoughts or trained beliefs as being simple, "*not to get emotionally involved in the patient's care. Empathy was more important than sympathy.*" Such a statement brings this thought to mind, "*how strange and hateful nurses are taught or learning to be.*" Most students were unaware that nobody cared. It took years for me to realize all that mattered was <u>income</u>.

Money for patient care from individuals and insurance companies provided salaries, and operating expenses. Many employees make up the staff in hospitals, convalescent homes, and long-term care facilities. There are aides, nurses, therapists, social workers, office workers, rehabilitation and occupational therapist; often assistants working privately for individual patients. Each requires a salary. Housekeeping departments also were part of the operating expenses, as was maintenance and grounds workers. Supplies are purchased with departments' allocation of funds, originating from taxation and contribution to the insurance companies, by yes indeed - those patients and their relatives. Other expenses in facilitates are for portable radiology equipment, linen services, and the list of miscellaneous equipment and other anticipated items. It goes on far longer than merely a paragraph or a page.

Honesty saves dollars and keeps facility costs down. Statistics detailing the cost of legal fees is an unexpected expense, often not allocated during a budgetary planning session; yet, when a patient disappears or suddenly is recorded as deceased - questions must be answered. For the average person it costs too much to get sick. One reality is socialized medicine; it works in several foreign countries. It has set a format of characterizations of wheels within wheels, turning but it cannot solely be looked upon as perfect, either.   There is no perfect way in which any facility or private caring household can deal with the consistent treatment required, to sustain life, in an identifiable style. Recuperating from an injury, allows a small percentile awareness, that needing others is far too costly than we all can afford. Without some sort of negative gut-feeling, truly, who is capable of knowing their care is adequate, with sufficient and helpful treatments, in an atmosphere of a decent location.

Negligence comes, varying in levels of minimal to gross; this brings fear into the public and private sectors' focus. Good treatment and medicines and personnel costs plenty. When does it not subside; reduce to an affordable level? Why after prepaying and contributing are many turned away, from care locally; being shifted midday in a crisis to a local or county facility has created trauma to patients. Frequently, transporting a patient has created forgetfulness with enhanced confusion, for youngsters and the elderly. These are makers of improvements for our technology in the future, with a long list of brilliant elderly that have contributed much advancement, throughout their lives and ours. Yet, each is being brought into a jungle of medical, surgical, and related-scientific dilemmas. It almost does not seem worth the time to complain, which is exactly what this book actually does. There have been times patients lashed out at nurses, doctors, housekeepers or the dietary staff. Not becoming angry by the treatments received: lack of concern, incorrectly prescribed medications with side effects, and causing drug-interactions as the major cause for violence (in the calmest and caring patients). Why...?

Indeed, why must such continue to be accepted after acknowledged reports, legal affirmations have proved malpractice, and expenses have been paid repeatedly? The answers that I have come up with would cause mighty discomfort, to administrative leadership in many facilities. In my opinion, employment would vest solely upon the emanation of facts; you do your job, you get paid. That seems simple; however, it also appears harsh, that the real world's cycle of capitalism, such occurrences happen. For every light or bell requesting comfort or help, medication, a journey to the lavatory - a dollar figure should be tacked on, to improve the service. How can I so arrogantly state my salvation, without considering the 'facts?' The facts are in my memories. I was there; I was observing. I did not forget both sides of the scenario I have complained about.

Because neglect depends on observations, it needs defining beyond the definition here. It also requires a balancing scale sorting out rights and wrongs. Neglect occurs and depends on the condition of patients or persons making a complaint, I have found. The involvement of those assuming patients' are being mistreated have plenty to do with legal aspects, which often follow when relatives or friends are believed to have become victims. The law views complaints as an important or useless balancing-scale. Some complaints are viewed as being maliciously, possibly pushed-aside till disregarded. Other complaints involve one or more attorneys, to prove neglect and define a remedy or settlement. Such legalities require approval of a judicial system, overwhelmed with murderers, thieves, technology hackers, and emotionally stressed with family problems.

Is there a place for medical feasible legal transformations in the United States? It has come and gone during the 1970s and 1980s, as far as I can see. There may never be any other malpractice nor facility citations negatively in my future, lest the continued care and desire by all scientists rebuild the image projected only to adolescents (as being, the blessed and perfect healers).

One sure way to commit to patient care, reduced abuses, and neglect was installing audio and visual equipment, in facilities. Telecommunication monitoring requires judicial approval, preventing an infringement upon 'human-rights' according to the first amendment freedom of speech! I ponder whether freedom of speech in a conspiracy to delve into a personal relationship at work, which prevents proper patient care is legal. That is neglect, often found in facilities; the more employees the greater this occurrence develops. And that is the one reason private facilities have become more popular; staff and management departments have stricter and enforced, patient care, forced upon the administration by public and judicial demands.

All forms of legal investigations add higher costs to the patients' care. Tacked on as: miscellaneous or other. Still, little can be ascertained by lay-persons, minimally aware of who the hell they are, let alone to wander about the halls of facilities filled with cover-ups.

Many improvements in facilities has occurred in the last two decades; actually, in the year 2003, it has increased over a three decade period of time. Students, volunteers, and medically assigned workers delved in deeply, brought facts and data regarding changes that surfaced, after many years of negative treatment. Eyes and ears of students, sees and hear things, some professionals overlook. Without infiltration of honest medically concerned students, reporting their views, neglect may have continued, at higher costs. Thus far medical treatment and care declining, from the neglectfulness once feared brings hopes back into the lives of the public.

For me, students with a desire to utilize standards of high-tech combined with patient care are better than brilliant intellectual linguists, speaking too educationally to me when I'm sick.

There is good treatment and poor, which has been already stated, in the above section one.

- Poor treatment is referred as neglectful.
- Care is hourly, daily, weekly, at home or in facilities.
- Long-term or permanent care has no structural of visible boundaries etched in stone; however, I truthfully saw such care can be altered, in a variety of ways, by employees awaiting salary versus genuine care. Therefore, it is essential for relatives and friends to combine their time, for visiting and participating in the care of loved-ones.
- Visitors decrease the negligence – by observing caregivers' - and reduces stress on the staff; it also improves the mentality of the infirmed.

Understanding the difference between long-term and intermittent has various definitions, as diagnosis of an illness for one patient may require a lengthy stay, and for others – just a brief stay in a facility. Accordingly, the injury or mental deficiency of an impaired, in conjunction to the visible concern, by the external community – all of which play a major roll in the road recovery. It does not single-handedly take a physician and staff workers; the healing process encompasses a wide range of individuals. Each concerned about proper treatments, care, and rehabilitation. In all my years of working and prying into several facilities, for personal knowledge, there is not much more that clearly defines the best facility. A varying patient care creates treatment, from facility to facility, rather than *'why is the sky blue with white clouds or purple and black overcasts, during rainstorms with lightning?'* So research local medical facilities, for yourself and loved ones. Ask questions and jot down answers, which are the expectations by your physician as acceptable. Insurance Companies mainly for the senior citizens care and treatment have websites, displaying statistics regarding facilities; medical staff and private physicians also carry a list of often unspoken preferential locations. Ask and ask again.

    Home care differs because there are no actual limits to treatments.

Portable equipment, ordered by a physician for patients to have X-Rays, blood tests, and rehabilitation therapy increases the cost to family.

Outpatient clinics and centers giving top-notch care and treatments, for patients physical and psychological well-being;, expensive as hell, not really.

Transportation has become less problematic with the introduction to public and private vehicles, transporting within local community; however, it is a service provided through homeowner and property taxed dollars. Currently, in this 21st century, medical centers offer patients transportation, to functions as a courtesy. This is a blessing. Obviously I should have inquired about who foots the expenses – medical center or patient insurance – but, I failed to think of asking before. It's as though we pay, pay more, and will continue to pay into programs and companies, for services that eventually may become unaffordable. This irks me because logically thinking, it cannot go beyond an imaginary *glass ceiling* without politicians and accounting firms going under.

Out Patient Services once were the least costly; many created clinical studies and care with limited but good formation, of available medical personnel, for non-critical ailments. Furthermore, these centers cost of overhead expenses have slowly escalated, nearly beyond affordability. Do such negative facts decrease or am I, and others continuing journeys into old-age without proper, expected, and deserved care?

Taber's Cyclopedic Medical Dictionary [edition 12] has many disease recognitions and definitions; includes are medical phrases, terminologies, linguistic dialogues and related data for aspiring students and professionals, desiring a complete knowledge enhancement during the 20th century. The book is old; not filled with the latest technology-advancements, the book was printed in 1973$^{©}$, not having many of the modern-day inclusions. Mostly there is numerous improvements and findings recorded, even though my book (Beware of Wolves in Sheep's Clothing) mentions negativity.

The Taber's book does have a utilization of intelligence, contributing emergency and first aid care, by not only medical or scientific students; it contributes tremendously, to nonprofessional as well. By the year 2000, it will definitely require a newer edition, for my collection of books; to enhance the available private knowledge, for a healthy living-experience, for those in my household. (2015 finds my book useful and has not been replaced, as I do not work in any medical field). Mostly in this modern day world of FOI (freedom of information) era information can be accessed online, through a variety of search engines; medical facilities and private medical centers provide 'portholes' for individuals to view their health related services.

There are sections outlining abbreviations, translations, and identification for body parts in their Latin and layperson terms. Although, it is not a book to read for personal gratification or relaxation, as a reference, periodically this 1975 edition of Taber's Encyclopedic Medical Dictionary did introduce and fulfilled its cost, many times over for me during my studies. Its estimated or average expectation for recovery patterns, often unknown, was flexible. The book included anticipative healing and recuperative time-spans, as guide-lines; making an ailment's improvement or decline, pathologically clear to perceive, as necessary to contact professionals when alternate methods seem to fail.

For instance: if the average somebody was told a child had a fractured collar bone, it would understood as being a broken neck...or would it? Some individuals do not understand the specific word variations of definition and sameness. Below are simple definitions of personnel frequently authorized to give or expected to give treatments to the injured, in various facilities or at home.

Attendants/Aides Attendants usually are male nursing assistants. Aides are female nursing assistants However, there are unisex gender interchanges with both titles. Primarily, males are physically more powerful or strong, compared to females; therefore, their strength for lifting and turning male or heavy bodies is far more needed than petite female aides. But, for time when there is no male assistant/attendant ... females learn to be independent and to utilize bed linens to aid during patient care alone..

Caretaker A parent, spouse, nurse or an undergraduate and adult adolescents are appointed as caretakers, to parents by a judge, at times...but, I often wonder why?

Concerned Family/Relatives There are either not enough or just too many. Sometimes, a patient needs to be away from overly caring or money hungry individuals to recuperate; to begin living again. Professionals usually have difficulty distinguishing those good from bad visitors; a concern usually ends up wasting the judicial system's time at high costs to the patient.

Nurse denied. One who cares for the sick, wounded or feeble, especially one who makes a profession of it, in a school of nursing? (according to Taber's)

Patient Injured individual or species; usually treated by physician approval, in one of a number of facility sites or home.

Physician A person who has successfully completed the prescribed course of studies in medicine within a medical school officially recognized by the country in which it is located, and who has acquired the requisite qualifications for licensing in the practice of medicine. (according to Taber's).

Proprietors Of Medical/Surgical Facilities. A Person or group as in a company [that] owns/operates one or more medical facilities where the injured are treated, cared for and given instruction on health related self-care. Basically, the personnel above work more than eight hour shifts. The non-registered and licensed nursing staff usually work between two to eight hours extra each week. Some work double-shifts more than twice a week.

> *An owner questioned my timecard for 90+ hours in a week, and 50 or more the next weeks - still to come. Little did the owner, facility administrative leader realize, nobody showed up for work many mornings; I didn't always remember to have the nurse in charge sign the timecard {many times I was exhausted, as I left to go home} I was asked to stay not because I was a registered nurse. No, I was required to stay at work because patients needed to be bathed, fed, have their soiled linen changed, etc. - and others did not show up for work.*

Students Taught to understand patients through role-playing. Mental exercise tends to reduce abuse and neglect. There are times when nothing taught can relieve a care-giver or care-taker of negative action or reaction toward one another. A good employee requirement consists of a standard practice, 'learn to eat, sleep, sleep, fart, shit, and hope to die,' for the job. As rude and arrogant that may be, it's the facts!

There are various departments giving treatment to patients, which depend on illness, disease, and faltering state-of-minds. Some patients may need surgery, others just a compress, often courtesy is one of the most needed but least received treatment of all!

Basically be aware-of minor things. If minor details are visibly neglected - how might the critical care be lacking, for starters. Is the facility prepared with twenty-four hour, a day resident physician, or physician assistant? Is the sufficient staff, consisting of both professionals and aids, technicians, and related employees to meet the needs of 'all patients?' You have to prepare for such things before illness appears. The list I shortened tremendously below could go on forever.

Emergency Treatment Differs greatly from permanent care. It is everything from care for a minor abrasion or laceration requiring a few sutures, to death or life threatening situations. EMTs of modern times see a variety of emergencies. Their jobs are to save lives and transport injured to an Emergency Room, for trained professionals to take charge. EMT training is intense. Practical and book learning are major requirements, for students to be responsible; a goal to work and feel special about the way they conduct themselves, on the job is essential. Hours on duty are far more than individuals believe. The field of EMTs consists of: First Rescue teams, Police Officers, Firemen [and fire-women] as well as community volunteers. Births are performed in ambulances en route to hospitals, Cab drivers as well have frequently transported emergency victims, delivered babies, and communicated for assistance from local police. It's not easy but its teamwork.

Pre-Op, Post-Op, Recovery Room This triad of careful treatment requires structured and detailed observation [plus] a specific treatment regimen.

Pre-Op means before an operation; also known as a surgical procedure. It includes special cleansing, with antiseptic and germicides; shaving the area to be repaired or explored, gathering of radiology films and necessary equipment for a surgical procedure to aid professionals before, during, and after the procedure. There isn't always advance time to gather physical research of patients' damage. Sometimes, life threatening situations require immediate surgery; specialists with either godly intelligence or an abundant experience ... prevent them from losing control under such pressures.

Post-Op A time of waiting for a patient to recover after a surgical procedure or critical time, the patient is observed either in the Operating Room (O.R.) or in a Recovery Room. Post-Op observations permit a clear view, of the recovering patient's current condition.   **Recovery Room** is where patients have monitoring of vitals signs begins, after surgical procedures and throughout the course of awakening, to be transported to an available hospital bed. In the recovery period usually, during critical surgery, monitoring is completely with technological equipment; however, O.R. Surgical Techs and Nurses continue to manually take vitals, and record changes. In critical surgical procedure such as open heart surgery, organ transplants, reconstructive skin grafts, patients are monitored, beyond opening their eyes and seemingly to be ready for transportation on a gurney to their assigned room.

Intensive Care Unit consists of a specialized team of professionals, to care for patients with seriously critical conditions; each patients is monitored in the ICU (Intensive Care Unit) every fifteen minutes. Monitoring, maintained by a specialized skilled nursing staff, trained in recuperative understandings. The team of specialists work long hours, many on-call for emergencies, around the clock. Recovery teams *are nurses, doctors, and technicians* are relied on by not only patients, they are as a family. As the patient is alert and coherent, returning to the room does not reduce nor stop monitoring; it merely reduces the times at which patients' vital signs are recorded. Data monitored and responses the patient displays are charted for the physician to analyze.

Births have special needs for both mom and infant The medical healthcare of moms set treatment apart from the newborn. The healthy mom usually presents no problem during the delivery; however, there are those trouble pregnancies whereby specialists are concerned for both the mother and baby, during and at the time of delivery. Typically, physical conditions of the mother such as: cardiac, respiratory, diabetic, and renal ailments create problem deliveries. More dangers occur in delivery rooms; drug-related births threaten the safety of both mother and newborn, by alcohol and/or illegal drug addictions. There are many purposes professionals turn a blind eye or deaf ear; unfortunately, a minority of patients created a vast cost increase through a personal lack of safety and self-preservational tactics.

Gynecologists and Obstetricians during the 1970 began refusing pregnant women; not because of prejudices or danger potentials at time of delivery. Malpractice suits of colleagues overpowered public media, leaving a fear within good doctors. Fears they would sue wrongfully, increased insurance costs, and created traumatic negative communications devastating many in the New England states. Pediatricians were often assigned when new mothers brought their newborn home, with little thought, or research. Somehow, I ponder - what's the use of worrying?!?

Gloomy realities may depress a reader, rather than enhance your self-analyst, to find your gut-feelings. Nothing is quite as simple as it may seem, especially in my book. Each case becomes a documentation, for physicians and nurses, to study. Everyone becomes a statistic when an accident occurs, during pregnancy and delivery of newborn, heart attacks, and other ailments are classified as statistics. Keeping your next occurrence in mind, consider yourself as a state to a high-priced caretaker or caregiver. You may reconsider going to the nearest local medical facility. Depending on related statistics to many conditions, illness may include a psychological intensity, not conducive to healing. Special needs required, by many patients with disabilities or those impaired with audio or visual deficiencies. If you are reading this book, be satisfied you have good vision; if it is not excellent at least you are not blind. They cannot see the faces of wrongdoers. The deaf cannot hear an attacker; many cannot speak for lack of listening to phonetics related to communication skills. Hmmm...! Yep, we that have five or that sixth sense - we are fortunate; we are blessed with abilities and functionalities a minor group have never known.

When patients, professionals, and private individuals analyze their lives and the income, changes take place. My dream is that medical facilities treat patients with 100% honest and proper techniques, for rapid recovery, to all. Realizing there will never be a 100% guaranteed skill-applied daily, I continue to include handicapped/disabled that have been neglected not merely by medical professionals for funds; they are more frequently abused by relatives and appointed care providers, often in their own home. Through research it can be statistically viewed, employees may complain about low wages, poor working conditions, and long shifts; how may are concerned with the care their patients are expecting, and paying for but not receiving? A chore most individuals cannot afford to do is worry needlessly over the lack in the funds which is probably more than many employees are worthy-of, from what I have personally encountered during the 1950s, 1960s (as a periodic patient); during the 1970s while training, I received negative facts on-site.

In the 1980s, more visits to neighbors, friends, and employment in the medical field gave way to additional updates. Unfortunately, after years of caring for others and being a concerned neighbor/friend, I found it a negative to work in a place of the non-caring individuals. One of my coworkers said, *"If a fire broke out I'd grab my purse and get the hell out of this place."*. Such a statement gave more truth to the average individual's thinking, as the patients are not important. How rotten…!

{1990s For me} Employment has since varied, to improve my image of my local community. Researching medical facilities had become my secondary passion; of which, I cannot change anyplace, for the better – at least not by myself. For true changes to improve care and treatment of patients, insurance companies and our government's legislation, permits, witnesses, and patients themselves must step forward. When someone's parent, child, or friend is believed to have received treatment or lack of care - that's when recording the situation must be brought to the attention of political leaders. Elected officials are representing the voters, and non-voters; therefore, permitting neglectful or harmful treatment should never be pushed aside.

It is politicians' responsibility to not only delve into community health issues, for which they represent the public. Wealthy or upper middle class incomes communities may be perfectly wonderful, on the surface; however, with offices out of reach by the average patient, politicians are often the last to receive information that is within their jurisdiction, to make note at meetings. They have the ability to create "Bills", to present verification of facts, and to request statutes be accepted into law, to remove negligence. And, to not only the wealthy but each and every individual, whether poor or paycheck to paycheck.

By keeping silent about complaints, the general public becomes far more damaged and filled with self-doubt; mainly because someone does not believe observations are or have been a mere oversight, and brushed under a stack of folders as clutter. Each oversight creates a situation that increases laxity, removing safety and essential common-courtesy and respect, from the only individuals that will become patients. So, standing still and quiet influences failures in professionals fields to not only ignore some; silence increases all related professionals to slack-off, in their area of specifics.

As difficult for employees to make a claim about negligence within the facility, it is also the responsibility of each to realize the harm, they too are permitting to continue. Understanding neglect comes in many ways; some clearly can be identified by visitors, others by professionals, and semi-educated in medical-surgical procedural care and treatment guidelines; students observe much more than the average visitor to a medical facility, and each minor unfilled patient call is a negligence. Each verbal and abuse from patients to the staff of decent professionals is also an abuse, and often goes untold, during shift changes; which also stands out as a minor event.

In all honesty, the call bell's button is for patients needing help immediately, not in a few minutes. Patients have understaffed floor nurses and aides, rarely are volunteer candy stripers available anymore. And as nightfall comes, the staff in many facilities becomes reduced from half a dozen to 2 or 3 per section; in one convalescent home, there was only

1 supervisor, 3 nurses, and 2 nursing aides/assistants caring for 50 patients. There many have been additional, however this was in the late 1970s and into the early 1980s.

It had improved somewhat, ratio nurse to patient in the 1990s; however, the shifts were increased from 8 hours to 12 daily, for 2 or 3 days with a day or two off.

Can anybody honestly claim all patients are requiring immediate help when the call button goes on? Absolutely not. There are actually, patients demanding immediate attention repeatedly; a few as the child that cries wolf once too often. That particular scenario is most likely the cost second of personal financial greed that has complicated malpractice suits. There are patients with demands that reek they are more important than somebody else. Nurses do not have the luxury of knowing at what moment the call button will be a truly necessary call for help. So, a mindful observation requires a critique of judgment, for both pesty patients and overworked nurses and staff.

What the hell is Proper Care or Treatment? It is difficult to reply straightforwardly without admitting, it depends upon the severity of the patient's ailment. In the studies of geriatric healthcare , during the mid-1970s, a class of approximately thirty students, including me, practiced under the supervision of a registered nurse; we studied diligently. Many interested in advancing for a nursing degree license continued on educationally. I was filled with too much, in personal obligations and responsibilities. Not that stating a fact of truth depleted my concern for the safety and well-being of patients, it merely pushed my curiosity higher.

My personal life was filled with raising my adolescents when not studying, and voluntarily applying my skills at work, to pursue a safe workplace. There was no time to consume lunches, coffee breaks, nor giggly-poo or just sitting around, doing my second choice in life, nothing at all; believe me, nothing at all is what I do now in this 21st century mostly. It's not as interesting as a young individual might believe. Of course, editing book length memories, inserting images and printing papers, does have me at a busy lifestyle after all. But, as a student back then - I, and many others, learned there were diverse patients. Some were unconscious, paralyzed, deranged, and violently abusive to anyone attempting assistance. Genuine test results were in patients' charts, for student to read and to retain data, during the care of assigned patients. 10 to 12 patients were assigned a nursing aide/assistant, in the morning shift. The afternoon shift had a decreased staff that led 20 to 25 patients get help from one aide/assistant. And the worse was that midnight shift; 2 nurse's aides/assistants per unit with 50 or more patients.

Reports by students as well as aides/assistants were entered, as nurse's notes, for physicians if any visited patients, to compare the improvement in condition. I rarely if ever seen a physician look in on any patients ,in the medical facilities (i.e.: nursing home, convalescent home, rehabilitation center). The course was training students to clinically input professionally, facts and events about patients; there was no time to train in "where are physicians". The equipment was excellent with sufficient machines, beds, wheelchairs, and professional daytime nursing staff. The afternoon till 11 pm staff was decreased with nurses have double case loads. The midnight till daytime shift, during training, students were not ever involved. However, I had personal employment experiences from previous nursing home and it was the worst shift, in many ways. Lack of more than two or three aids per thirty to forty patient-counts was unfair, intolerable, and at times, allowed minimal care to patients confined to beds. As a student there was a completely different aspect of nursing projected; it consisted of bedridden patients receiving bed baths with two nurses, tray feedings for those unable to sit in wheelchairs, and physically walking weak patients to the lavatory. Assigned care diversely varied between male and females patients. Frequently, male nurses (attendants, orderlies, and assistants) were assigned the heavy males that were unable to physically move about without at least two people's help. Several good male nursing students dropped of the course, for lack of concern by the staff.

Daily Care face and hand washings, dentures brushed, rinsed, and placed in patient's mouth, dressing the patients in clean hospital gowns were chores, for one worker assigned ten to fifteen patients. Bed making with mitered corners, to prevent decubitus to bedridden patients, and for comfort to those wanting to lay down for a nap was consistent of a single-workers (assigned patients) daily. As boring and beneath us as that may seem it was essential for good patient care.

Daily Nourishment was served to many patient's in a dining room; others remained in bed with a mobile tray. A few patients required nurse's help to cut and eat foods, to remove lids, and to drink from a straw. Many were unaccustomed to eating three meals a day with a snack. Others could not walk to the dining room; they were in placed in wheelchairs, tied with a 'pull-sheet', so they would not slip onto the floor during dining, at a table with others. Usually, patients under sedation or not on a special diet require less care. They were a blessing.

Rest/Sleep day or night required most patients was a regime of precautionary preventive care, from self inflicting injuries. As one would protect a newborn, so was it necessary to protect patients in their 80s, 90s, and beyond from scratching, and rolling out of bed; restraints were applied to wrists normally. Patients with psychological disorders or medicated became disoriented and hostile, being jostled about, by nurses or aides.

At times, frail patients during the daytime were tied with restraints, in wheelchairs, to preventive self harm. A majority of patients in nursing homes, convalescent homes, and rehabilitation centers required full care. Many unable to leave their bed, to evacuate feces or urine; they required immediate assistance to the lavatory. Unfortunately, even I had found several patients truly were ringing for a nurse {because} they were lonely. Those patients created an element/atmosphere of pestering the staff periodically.

Although, it is essential for patients to become mentally aware or relieved of their discomforts, visible or internal, the prescriptions authorized by physicians at the entrance to a facility is not changed; leading patients and staff responsibility totally to the facility. Patients did not get followed up appointments, in long-term facilities; patients seemed to be set-aside as in '_never-never-land._'

During the 20th century massive malpractice suits were encountered and conveyed to the public, in public broadcasts. There were only a small percent of changes, for legal actions; primarily toward the 1990s, there were major improvements that I personally have observed. The care and treatment during a life threatening ailment, of a respiratory ailment, mild heart attack brought me to the emergency. Transported by EMTs most certainly gave me another wake-up call. For the first time in my life other patients and me had something in common; fear, yes plain and simple *FEAR*.

I was scared, believing I'd be left to die by an understaffed hospital; much to my surprise, I was treated as though I had been a major financial contributor, as though I might have been somebody of great importance. This was a tremendous get well momentum that should never go unmentioned.

Equipment monitored vital signs. The nurses and doctors, and the aides were the most heartwarming and compassionate beings I could have ever anticipated, to find in a local hospital. They transported me to radiology with care, concern, and I was not left alone to think: *"what the hell was going to occur if I could not catch my breath;"* a radiology technician performed their job. A nursing aide was there, comforting me, which is a mental need, during any crisis. And once admitted to a room, monitoring continued; nothing I did was unknown to the 'Nurse's Station' amazing.

I wrote a letter to the administrative leadership, commended the staff from a majority of levels that I found to be superb. For me to mention improvements, it is the real-thing, because I am judgmental, as this book clearly states. I have been told that medical professionals in or out of their field are the worst patients; yes, it is absolutely true. A patient with a background at any level in medical/scientific levels critiques down to the very smallest negativity.

Volunteers do not get paid; each provides a time span of 1 hour to several, daily. Many are senior citizens, as well as students and candy stripers, in the 20th century. Some received free lunches, and discounts on medical care. Students became disgusted by conditions, as volunteers were never permitted to actually adjust a patient's bed, fluff a pillow, or escort patients to the lavatory. A volunteer was permitted to read, write a memo, answer the telephone, and call for the nurse. Complaints came to the attention of administrative officers, regarding protocol for logical safety, and beneficial use or needs of volunteers. Volunteers were permitted back then to read correspondence, distribute newspapers to patients interested in community or global affairs.

Psyche wards for psychologically impaired, required professional licensed personnel with both educational and physical strengths. Somehow, I would not have been of much use, in such an atmosphere. Many nurses were under direct physician-orders in patient care. How sad, to find, in order to receive long-term care properly during the 20th century, patients had to be diagnosed as mentally malfunctioning or deficient? Yuck...!

I remember supervisors, in medical facilities, did not wish to associate or communicate with assistants or aides; as though they were less important than the licensed professionals. Supervisors and Charge Nurses communicated with RNs and LPNs because of status levels. The level of major patient care, consisted of administering injections, tablets, liquids, applications of salves and bandage changing, and numerous other prescribed treatments, by a physician. Intravenous (IV) care, Gavage (tube) feedings, and Catheter care was restricted to nurses. Nurses were responsible for starting and monitoring blood transfusions, which I have found most recently has become the responsibility of medical assistants and laboratory technicians. The medical field has made many errors, which most have been improved upon to a nearly perfect level.

Yes, there has been immeasurable break throughs, of excellence; technologically has opened the doors to improved and accurate monitoring, observation, and treatments. And, since the earliest community care centers were developed/opened, in the late 19th century truly beneficial administering of medications and over-all patient healing has focused upon improvement, after improvement. The need for improvement not only in the medical field but in many other field, stands to gain by joint-efforts and endeavors of both professionals and students.

To reiterate *students* create inquiries often to problems that can be adjusted or improved upon with modern technologies. Not all students. Only a mere handful face a fully concern, in care of the infirmed. But those are the few that dedicate their lives to making health not only a professional field but a lifelong career, to be proud of.

From my point of view there has been no great improvement during the 1970s, as a layperson; however, as a patient and low-level experienced caregiver, I visibly have observed advancements in equipment to detect complications, chronic or recurring methods of diagnostics machines, and many more refined and alert personnel increasingly catering genuinely to patients.

Communities with many elderly, have a better change of receiving modern technologies than a youthful population. Needs differ in age levels, incomes and insurances vary, so do ailments in physical and psychological aspects. Facts and statistics will be available only as reported situations, of negative and/or positive occurrences become documented; and it is easy to locate on the Internet comparable facts and figures, by geographic locations. Often too realistic than many individuals would believe, comparing locations' healthcare displays probable ailments are endemic.

Actuaries provide and utilize statistics in diverse rate changes. Accountants utilize annual percent and cost of living increases by the previous year, and years prior. Statistics are important but many valuable statistics can be accessed, by those interested enough to seek recorded facts. Insurance companies use actuarial data before providing whole life insurance, health insurance, vehicle insurance, and home-owners insurance; statistics include in the query: race, age, health, location, activity, and income. Yep there is probably much more in an actuary, which interested individuals will benefit from viewing.

Much to my surprise, malpractice legal actions once a final judgment has been documented, by justice system is available to the public. Knowing the percent of claims against a facility, professional, or legal system avails critical data, for both statistical references, and where to go when ailments arise could depend on your knowledge.

I always thought of a time when I would have a few dollars to go to a movie, eat popcorn or candy, and drink a soda during my youth; when I wouldn't be depleting my monthly funds, it seemed each want did not benefit anything more than a few hours of screen viewing. I think I'm just about at that point in my life, when finances of my future is an major-concern; perhaps that is why I am writing recollections of miserable job-related facilities. During that second half of the 20th century, I hated my job(s); many other individuals hated their jobs too.

Numerous individuals did not feel anger or hate, for their jobs because of the work but the lack of concern, by employers. I was informed if I did not like the standard of upper managerial expectations, I was free to quit. That truly was not what I would have expected, to hear during a dilemma of moral and ethical opinions and personal views. When I did quit, I was called back to work; there were limited employees willing to pull double shifts, at minimum wage two or three days a week. As for myself, I expected my salary no matter what, as patient care was provided properly by me and those aides I worked closely with.

The employers cared little of employees waiting for buses, in the darkness of night. I, personally, walked to work frequently because buses did not run regularly, at a time when I needed one. My funds were limited to rent, food, clothing, and bare-essentials. Guess I should be ashamed or embarrassed to admit I hated being an aide with a good attitude, and thoughtfulness towards patients while upper level personnel conveyed snide remarks, about how pesty numerous patients were!

There is more to working in facilities than movies such as **One Flew Over the Cuckoo's Nest** and **On Golden Pond.** Those two movies convey realities that I believe prompted investigations, into poor care, in not only the elderly and long-term facilities. Those movies conveyed some individuals were confined against their will. Others lived in solitude, to survive external elements that contributed to permanent confinement. Both movies inform the public of several irregularities, depicting low income City hospital's problems, as well as minimal staff and overcrowded wards. The concern of staff for confined patients with psychological disorders is similar to the movie's disclosures, in some instances where incorrect diagnoses have prevented proper medications to improve and possibly cure, ailing momentarily disgusted individuals. In the real world, medical facilities find patients as being a threat not to one another but to the system. Their

44

intellect can bring light to shock, stress, and damage mistruths, about treatment or lack of good care. Patients with physical or psychological disorders rarely are availed opportunities to confer with physicians or attorneys; for many patients, connection to the outside world is practically nil! Conveyed facts, of mistreatments create doubt of professionals that eventually will require care, yet somehow rare is it that professionally look in the future, to how they will be treated.

The movie **On Golden Pond,** I viewed two or three times; truly it touched me in a spiritual and psychological way. I cried through most of the movie, the first viewing. It made me more aware of how awful the world could be [probably do to my experience as a medical facility employee]. Ups-and-downs of living with or without a fair mental standing surfaced as Katharine Hepburn and Henry Fonda portrayed the life-style, of an aged couple, alone in a cabin overlooking a lake. He with dementia or stages of Alzheimer's disease gave the public something to associate with, as we too are susceptible. Several months, perhaps a year later the movie appeared on television; I felt saddened again, observing the future for myself and millions of others.

Patient care and treatment not only dictates attempting to produce a good end-result, it also entails care and reporting an accident, in a facility. When a patient falls out of bed, slips in a bathroom or shower, there were times no physicians were available, to examine the incident; a report was written by an available Supervisor, Head Nurses, or Charge Nurse. Mostly the incident report included how the patient looked, asking simple things to see if the patient responded coherently. If the observation revealed nothing more than a bruise with patient(s) seeming to be coherent, a written accident report followed. The next day, a physician (if one was on file, in the patient's chart) was notified. For possible serious injury, emergency treatment was started, reluctantly. There were times a patient was sent by ambulance to hospital emergency rooms, to a nearby hospital. Most patients in long-term care facilities have trouble standing without assistance, not because of an injury but they were frail with brittle bones; others were sedated to the point of incoherency, from physical ailments.

There were so many ailments classified as being terminal; many could have been reversed. Who am I to consider writing about such a topic? Nobody more than myself, a former nursing aide. Terminal means there is no hope of recovery, from an illness but it is also an allocation of verbiage, to convey to elderly that are no longer able to live on their own. Patients in long term facilities have a duration leading to doom. Family relatives and friends can do nothing or so they chose. Some just do not car at all. The reason is plain and simple, it requires time, money, and allocation of a room for the aging person. Some patients require special apparatus, for safety co-efficiency. Others require electronic equipment can be rented or purchased, at expensive costs, when insurance does not provide funds. In addition to at home care verses medical facility care often is weighed by analyzing the costs of visiting nurses, aides, homemakers, and physicians care, which frequently requires physically transporting a patient periodically to an office. A long list of professionals have greatly improved, in lieu of financial concerns when physicians approve insurance expectations to cover Social Workers, Therapists, and Laboratory Technicians to complete documentation to avail analytical input, to provide a prognosis. However, physicians that care about the improved private care, in relative homes or condominiums create high-insurance premiums. I wonder if it's worth the living experience, to grow to old-age after all this information is conveyed?

Communities developing centers or programs coinciding to high schools have increased the safety to many elderly or confined, to a private dwelling place; their visits, reports, and sometimes just their friendly attitude, supports the emotional needs, often overlooked by professionals. Benefits from the community, not only encourages individuals to want to live, it develops additional input for increased techniques, for future creations to make aging, easier. It seems healthcare has become the number concern not only for those mature, ailing, for students looking forward to promoting a reduced stress, as they to build their lives.

From personal observation in the 1970s I recall amputee patients with prosthetics as miserable, physically, by ill-fitted legs. Colostomy patients embarrassed, by a nurse having to assist change a bag, to cleanse the area, of fecal-matter. Nursing assistants, aides, orderlies, and each level of licensed nursing staff requires patient full-care; however, the higher up your career the less of the patient cleansing, is required. With licensing responsibility increases; questions I ask myself: "how come, why, and various related questions" as to " ...*each licensed nurse, doctor, and technician must have a mentality of non-responsibility?*"

There would not be minimal-to-massive patient abuses, if staff members developed an agenda correctly, during training. Compassion and empathy would have continued throughout increased educational pursuits. Somehow, in many occurrences it has been 'negative attitudes,' seeking perfection.

Prosthetics and **implants** have been improved upon, for patients requiring replacements of teeth, extremities, and organs. Perhaps the best surgical procedures have been the most visibly grotesque historically. More currently, media impact 'talk-show' hosts and newscasters and commentators brought prosthetics, and surgical replacements into the public view. Patients verbalizing their experiences of daily living. Frequently, many do not convey experiences in a physician's office, hospital, and that extremely recuperative period of time, noted as recovery and occupational therapy sessions keeps silenced truthfulness.

During physical and/or occupational rehabilitation, patients suffer tremendous physical and psychological stress; complaints, remarks, and emotional feelings seldom are revealed. That silence contributes to neglect in a path of solitude. "*Silence is golden*," my dad would say, during an argument or oral dispute with my mother. The way to face reality as my life continued, followed that path; writing memos to myself, and that attitude and belief is what led to creating this book of babbling-on, and on, and on. Yes although I have my total body parts, there are horrible scars that make me feel inferior as well as rejected by others at times. So too are individuals with prosthetics; not out of psychological self-betrayal. These individuals being taught to accept what is not there any longer, to accept artificial limbs, and to accept that asshole individuals will jeer them.

A valuable lesson learned, whether intentionally taught or not, *it's not easy being mutilated; prosthetics may have eased patients with a handicap into being capable of serving themselves, and not being totally depended on others*.' The facts on the other side of the coin convey outrage, patients incurred; not by self-pity. Many patients muttering ohw's and o's during procedures being consoled, by a nurse or attendant, as others peer sympathetically.

As when having a Dentist give an injection of **Novocain** prior to oral surgery, it is a widely used to numb an area (i.e.: jaws, gums, and open wounds to be sutured). Unfortunately, the affect wears off, leaving not only patients with physical scars but emotional pain, far beyond any prescription medicine. Long, regularly scheduled sessions with professional counselors may reduce stress through verbal expression. Patients do not often receive financing for their additional sessions required. Nor do insurance companies divvy out any new prospective future plan, for the patient requiring resizing of a prosthetic or implant, as their body grows or with age. Does it sound as if I hate the medical and surgical world's brilliance? In a small way, I do. In another way, I think what a rotten and evil world it would be, had modern medicine's world of experimentation stopped progressing.

Babies born with no limps, Siamese twins (attached; and detached surgically), and an extremity injured requiring removal to, save somebody's life. Such realistic overviews, make some surgical procedures an asset, at times. Rejoining a digit sliced off by a child during bicycle exploring of the metal chain; cranial, facial, and other body scars reduced, to publicly accepted viewing, by reconstructive surgical procedures have proven to be healing factors. All I truly have to complaint about is patients living with psychological pressures/stressfulness attempting to survive the future with adjustments, physically and emotionally, why are they not cared-for with dignity? Why are they not looked upon as an injured being rather than a freak?

*"How come they are bilked out of thousands to billions of dollars (*of public, private, and insurance *funding. Furthermore when does the personal injury of one, to hundreds-of-millions stop, from violent weaponry as in war-time?"*

I am ending this chapter "Patient Treatment" with a final question; "*Has humanity became so inhumane; permitting personal and professional greed to lead to violence, in order to maintain imagines, of responsible-beings 'hard-at-work'?"*

Let me not damage the medical industry or field anymore than already done, in previous chapters. The previous chapter stated assorted care a patient should be able to expect, that they actually should receive. It includes: cleanliness, personal grooming, dining or being fed, occasional midday or evening snacks (would be nice as well), and common courtesy with an air of professionalism. Of course, there has been and will most likely continue to be 'a hand of patients' truly, **nutso**! For them, saintly medical teams are provided with sedatives, to minimize outbursts by both male and female patients. In basic daily medical facilities, the handful of rotten, nasty, violent patients do not compliment the job, in any way, of the staff in any area of employment. The medical field however is trained from day one, how to cope with negative patients. On the whole, patients wish to be treated better than they would expect by those being provided salaries, from their family or friends.

This makes sense to me. Taxes pay for medical care, insurance companies pay facilities for medical care, and patients, as well as 'potential' patients, provide the premiums. "*Am I wrong?*" Well, the way I see it, all people, including: the homeless, bums, thugs, workaholics, and all other sweet-darlings provide at one time or another, incomes to others for proper and kindness; their monies are contributions to the medical facilities and insurance companies, in daily employment deductions, quite often. So, again, "why have I and many others viewed negligence and rarely reporting incidents, to local authorities as complaints, hopefully to minimize further occurrences?" Me, I am baffled; I have no-idea why keeping silent would be less emotionally rewarding than speaking out. for a better way. The research in this book comes not only from my observations.

Some observations I reported, were ignored, by facility staff and upper management. Political municipal and state representatives that I have written, informing them that they need to delve into horrendous or minor but negative conditions, conveyed "thank you correspondence" to me. Decade after decade new investigative companies are incorporating ideas as well as individually prying into complaints; many actually have that 'big brother is watching you' intimidatingly, placing the fear of God, Allah, or be damned Satanic worshippers till improvements have been made. Prying public and private sectors have me satisfied, knowing I can complain, or brag, as I or others view progressive change.

Progressive change includes reduced stress and pain. Progressive change creates occupation, rehabilitation & recuperation in therapeutic centers more increased safety and well-being without depleting care from: <u>personal, private, and public funds nearly as much as neglect increases such activities</u>.

To cut this paragraph short: "<u>abuses whether accidental or intentionally caused, by neglect,</u>" require a good set of sense to detection. A few detection questions include:

<u>Observations of patient in bed, chair, lavatory, and obvious signs to the nurse?</u>

1. Is patient's bed clean and free of crumpling?
2. Are bed linens, pillows, blankets, and patient gown free of massive wrinkles?
3. Has patient been properly propped in bed?
4. Do patient's feet touch foot board?
5. Has patient's bedding filled with cluttering papers, periodicals, food or crumbs, blood stains, urine, feces, and/or vomit?
6. Are intravenous tubes dislodged, displaying blood, or not dripping in tubing?
7. Has a foul odor filled patient's room?
8. Is climate control functioning, to maintain temperature comfortably?
9. Do the patient have a HELP remote within reach?
10. Are drainage tubes, after surgery requiring attention, do to a discharge or bloody wound area?
11. Mainly does patient communicate sufficiently, in language of facility?
12. Are there signs of senility, Alzheimer disease, irrationalism, and/or reduced cognition?
13. Are patient needs primarily non assisted or requiring a private assistant?

Because patient needs and patient requirements en route to recovery differ, as much as one disease to another, an assessment is necessary at admission, to a medical facility. Monitoring vital signs, healing process, and patients ability to independently function should be noted with care, by a registered nurse, **first**. Thereafter, a licensed practical nurse, and a nurse's aide or assistant can convey observations – to expedite a comparable analysis. Using professional guidelines, on the first day a patient is admitted to a facility creates a flow of properly set forth routines; in addition, decreased abuse can be readily promoted.

Both non-abusive and abusive individuals require good instincts, for self preservation. The neglectful must stay on-top of their actions, to cover the faults; victims are less protected, by themselves, in medical facilities. The patient needs witnesses to prosecute. This almost does not make sense because individuals with normal mental capacity do not intentionally cast-ill-remarks/false allegations. Gut-feeling is mostly what parents refer to when having mature conversations or giving lectures - to their kids. To a patient that same type of calm but straightforward talk gets the facts surfaced. Ask the questions above; not necessarily all. Ask what appears to be told.

Throw in questions of your own, such as:
1. "Have you been seen by your doctor?"
2. "Did you go to the bathroom with or without a nurse?"
3. "What did you eat earlier?"
4. "Are you in any pain or discomfort?"

say something, like: "go with your gut feeling. If you think its wrong, don't do it." A few known senses are listed below. Senses can provide information about a patient's care. During a patient's stay in a medical facility their observations of surroundings outside the room can create additional questions regarding care and treatment. Noticing the staff walking about from room to room, housekeepers working, dietary distributing trays, and other patients ambulating with or without assistance increases a low to no abusive facility. So here goes.

- **Instinct** can be the first and firmest selective criteria, in any daily activity. Gut-feeling is normally a jittery uncertainty prior to attempting challenges. Butterflies in the stomach marks many a nervous moment, attempting something for the first time. Goosebumps when an eeriness creeps up without noticeable signs.

- **Sight** with it you can see your enemy or best friend, and what is in or passed your path. *Your eyes are only one warning signal.* They are not merely the window to the soul!

- **Hearing** it is not easy to detect *all noises or sounds.* It takes practice to know a tone and the level of rhythmic noise as it is related in a familiar way to something. Adolescents frequently recognize the telephone ring, doorbell chimes, and the voice tones' of their parents and educators, both during comfortable speech and harsh, as when they are being reprimanded. It takes practice to identify melody orchestrations. Howls differ from a wild dog to that of a house-broken pet. Cats, are not easily identified according to age, by voice tones lest listening has become a standard for mentally alerting one's self what the animal is conveying. Even newborns have a diverse crying pattern; each gurgle as well conveys something is either quite right or absolutely turning into a negative situation. So taking the time to listen, hear and practically study noise, can only improve the safety and well being of not one person; such studies whether professionally in universities or independently, for personal knowledge can save your life. Identifying sounds can be a utilization tool for developing facts, in criminal or civil judicial proceedings.

- **Touch** natural instincts acquired at birth, according to numerous pediatricians and numerous psychologists; even grandparents have a tendency to refer to touch, as a baby's basic need. Items such as: *word, stone, skin, fur, paper, plastic, cloth, clay, wool, metal, and textures* more diverse as modern technologies create better more durable products, increase human knowledge. Textures can identify an attacker's clothing, skin, or weapon. I find myself during a shopping spree or browsing through department stores – touching a fabric, ceramic ornament, and other items before purchasing. Why? It has become a habit since my childhood when I lost vision in one eye.

o **Smell** yep, it _really sticks_ when you pay money to insurance companies, governing powers only to find in your time of treatment for many injuries, professionals are nothing more than financial wizards, with your money. _Aside from that amusing memo_ the real truth, consists of: _fragrances_ that surround us throughout our lifetimes. The air we breathe may not have a smell you recognize till you enter a room of smoke. Fog may not have a distinct smell but flowers, shrubs, vegetables, and fruits – most certainly do. Recognizing _smells, scents, aromas, fragrances or nothing at all_ can be identified within your nostrils in a negative or positive function. Your mind leads you to safety from nasty odors. Your mind prevents you from leaving a positively, fragrant area … for a minute or two longer than you'd have been prepared to remain. Fragrance has created a few legal proceedings definite convictions, by blind witnesses, testifying during a trial. Therefore, it is good to know numerous odors can either identify you or an assailant, use of similar fragrances distinguish you from me, and other from millions of other people, at times, even applying exact scents, to different bodies. Having something to do with the body temperature, combination of fabric material and applied fragrance may differ. However, basic fragrances of farming produce, floral arrangements, and musty odors that are unpleasant – many will:

o **Taste** Foods are valued expressions of caring; mothers serve or offer sweets during a momentarily crisis to adolescents or loved-ones. More often than I care to admit, many mothers including me, eat cake, pie, cookies, or drink sweet beverages during turmoil. There seems to be an elegant, sedateness naturally brought to the surface during negative moments, by ingesting decadent stuff. Fathers, boyfriends, and numerous top-notch males prefer a liquor beverage after a full day's work, filled with horrid or unpleasant experiences; beer, wine, martinis and a slue of other – considerably detrimental ingestible products, sooth their weariness before their journey home. Often enough there are murders from otherwise soothing products, by unsuspected villains. Deaths from poisonous products, have become medically detectable through much research, and autopsies. However, using one's senses/instincts prior to consuming products will realistically prevent many severe, harmful incidents.

Our six senses may seem ignorantly depicted, in an alarming way; however, the basic senses are instinctually the body's compass, for safe direction, in any given place or time. Furthermore, studies in universities such as NOVA Southeastern in Florida, and many more colleges around the world contributions of medical and technology learned observations of animal research, which has led major improvements. Improvements that might not have proved man and animal life share natural instincts. Both man and beast share natural instincts to <u>herbaceous</u>, <u>cavernous</u>, and <u>omnivorous reproductions</u>, for nourishment.

Simply enter a garden center, observe plant-life; select two or several species of plants. Bringing your selections home, set aside a time, a day for journalizing, the growth, and development of each plant and its variations. Amazements will surface. A floral may sprout numerous buds, fragrance, and re-fertilize its soil. Foliage may not seem to reproduce a leave or new stem for many weeks, or months. Out of the blue an unbelievable and abundant development appears.

Things are different in development just as human beings and beast vary. What does plant and animal life have to do with human beings? Plenty.

As the weather chills, observations will view changes:

- **humans** cover up with sweaters, jackets, socks, and closed shoes or boots.

As the climate intensifies heat-wise in summer:

- less clothing is worn; more beverages served over ice is consumed.

Now, compare yourself to plants and animals. Take a look at a documentary, on a travel channel; notice the fur on wild animals.

- Hardy firm stems with leaves become vibrant in springtime but in summer wilted.

- During the summer the fur becomes thinned. Animals reduce in body weight because the heat reducing the appetite.

- Plants in autumn and winter gain instinctual temperatures, by developing leaves for warmth, and dormancy occurs that decreases growth of fruit, vegetation, or flowers.

- Animal in winter display a complete opposite effect. Skin and fur becomes thicker, appetites increase, weight gain and tiredness occurs; this is a way of body's instinctual protection against harsh cold weather.

As with varying living things, I have observed neutrality, in vibrant diverse revelations when it comes down to, *"the norm!"* And to top this lengthy set of *instinctual-navigation elements* within all beings, in my childhood, I had been informed with the loss of one 'sense' instincts each have an enhancement, strengthening as instinctual compensation.

"Does that seem like a bunch of crap?

Yes, but it is not!" Practice of 'awareness tests' took place; each supervised between two or more individuals, by professional. as the visual preceptors, speakers, listeners, smellers, tasters, apparently the expectations in diagnostic responses were compared to numerous other answers. Eventually the compared findings were evaluated and journalized, for future references. Perhaps, that simple but complete examination created my instinct to practice observations on my own. And, then again, my natural instincts have utilized other diversities, in writing this book and quite a few others, on different topics. Am I pleased that I was a guinea-pig? Absolutely not! Do I feel my privacy was infringed upon? One hundred percent! And, furthermore, because I was injured leaving lifelong scars, I was categorized as handicapped; a stigmatizing title which created an emotional and harmful pathologic road of nearly-doom.

Personal endeavors, fighting the system of perfect students' in public schooling, and selecting occupations of persistent downfalls was my recourse; growth and development, for me, was judged upon not my ability but the diagnostic results posted in a file. Fortunately, that negative and incorrectly monitored file has become obsolete. I have achieved, only when it was important for me to be accepted. My goals were often opposite of educators, leaderships, and clergy beliefs. My mind delves beyond the visual and audio perceived observations taught in communities, to stress personal and community camaraderie. My values stems from the early start I have had in the 1950s, by a majority of scientific mentalities, often neglectful towards handicapped, feeble, senile, and selected guinea-pig parents could not understand. In a way, my downfall's beginning was an *obstruction-of-justice* [for me] forcing me to focus on a pathology, of my own capacity and interests.

- How might you, the readers, know when an abuse is intentional or accidental?
- Where would your observation be reported, for immediate or any impact, at all?
- Why should you probe into the facility a friend or relative enters, for treatment?"
- If you were infirmed, neglected, abused, or left to actually urine, vomit, or evaluate your bowels, and lay in the soiled bed-linens, for more than five minutes, what process would you once well follow?

Keeping that disgusting but factual question and answer section in the back of you mind, reading this book my not be as important. You know have the ability to realize or rationalize my purpose for writing such gory, seemingly nonsense. You can continue to read this book if you have a difference opinion, and you may even find your money … you know financial contributions, to prevent carelessness is a waste of time without verifiable documentation of complaints.

We all have visited a hospital when a new baby is born, to a friend, spouse, relative or even a close neighbor. There are two observations to look for, at that time. One is for the safety and well being of the baby, in a Nursery with several other newborns. Peek at the floor and walls; is there drywall falling of peeling wall-coverings in clear view? Are babies screaming with not a glimpse of a nurse or other attendant? Are soiled cradle linens bunched up in over-stuffed bins or is garbage bins filled to the maximum capacity? Glance at each baby. Yes, they are adorable. I know!

But, are they safe? Do any appear discolored? Maybe there are markings of a bruise or needles with tubes inserted to the cranium. Do you think it's necessary? If not, ask one of those nurses that transports your patient's newborn, what's with that baby with those tubes or needles or bruises? Many individuals would not have the balls to inquiry. Many individuals do not view others as being important enough. Unfortunately, those considered to be '*less important enough to us today*', may have significant value, to our future or the future of complete strangers. Maybe everyone should delve into their souls; that silent but invisible conscience. Answers lie there and we seldom take a minute to seek.

Most of us, including myself more often than I should convey, figure … '*hey, myself, my spouse, my kids, their spouses and kids, and the few surroundings I developed - such as a faltering garden, pet-domestic-haven which should be left to professional pet caregivers, and such trivial personal cares take too much time than to consider others …!*' However, the newborns get each of our hearts filled with warmth, compassion, and inborn nurturing flows. SO, now look at the patient room. Is it horrendous? Bed linens though messy are not neglectful symptoms of a bad staff. It could mean you are visiting a person that tosses and turns. Negligence is spills from a water jug, urine, or blood on the floor for long periods of time. Side-rails down on both sides of a bed, as a sedated or sleeping patient are unattended. Loud music or televised programs blaring, annoying but remaining after a request or two has been brought to the attention of staff, that ignore it. Empty intravenous or blood bottles (or plastic bags) hanging from IV poles, for more than an hour. Even an hour is too long. Professional care should be rapid, yesterday when ever possible, with no ignoring or snide slurring beneath the breath of the nurse or staff members.

Housekeeping is not responsible for cleansing or clearing away: *intravenous feeding equipment, patient food trays or water jugs*, and certainly that department does not have an obligation to care for patients. Quite frequently these are alert and caring individuals; often overlooked by visitors, patients, and medical personnel. Many of the chores for maintenance and housekeeping is considered menial. Somehow, there would be no linens, towels, gowns, and certainly not a fixture in properly working order had there been no employees working, for improvements and appearances of both patient rooms and the entire facility.

As important and basic as signing a consent form during a crisis can authorize surgical procedures; malpractice litigations continue with such, for years, before a final judgment or legislation can be added/removed from the patient rights. Of course, animal and plant rights have wildly spread rumors of becoming valuable; many complaints are often overlooked, cast aside, and dealt with as if each was a pestering occurrences. It seems to me, once rights are infringed upon negatively to a species, the life foyer gets filled with unacceptable, repeated annoyances. No matter what the terminology refers to when complaints are left in file cabinets, changes cannot be accomplished.

Volunteers, freely function assisting patients write and read correspondence, rather than be recognized as entrusted to develop or assist. Verbally executives or staff members in an occupation or profession with body-language constitutes fraudulent concerns, as looking downwardly on volunteers.

Necessary steps must be ascertained, to utilize and to accept free help, for improved healthcare as well as within other non-medical fields. Suggestions are only as good as the listeners perceive I have come to believe, yet filed away complaints, remedies, and verbal accusations often go without any recognition or viewing at all.

Can such atrocities be prevented or stopped? Will executives ever face their dilemma of loss in business, income, or reliable associations? These two very important questions are truly worthy of individuals privately seeking to improve their working conditions, and including future prospective clients, patients, and related communications – to reinvent the wheel so to speak. A company is created or incorporated to bring more business. Without satisfied customers and consumers there is no future business. It's that simple. Be good to the individuals you are caring or serving; and that normal chain of action and reaction from them will provide an increase to your beginning goal to make or serve a product to earn an income. There is nothing threatening, nor degrading about being decent to consumers. Consumers need medical/surgical/dental/psychological and other help. Nobody can do everything themselves. If they can, well, I wish I could meet those perfectly brilliant folks.

In a nutshell, the complete opposition to the ***Hippocratic Oath*** doctors swear to uphold has been degraded and ignored many times repeatedly, by mature and responsible individuals that *once* accepted it. Not only must something be done to protect patients; I believe legally, that oath should be analyzed, with addendums or inclusions, to create a more concisely written document of moral and professional conformity. But, as an individual, I stand unanimously singled-out in a vast field of concern, too costly for anything to be taken less seriously.

Agencies, organizations, foundations, societies, and government committees formed during three centuries when patient care and treatment was deemed inhumane. However, in the earliest years of medical treatments, reduction of pain during removal of teeth, limps, and suturing merely skimmed the surface of where and how to decrease anguish, bodily and mental injury to was encountered.

- In the 19th century community groups formed
- In the 20th century agencies and committees developed standards, frequently monitored amongst the best to worst facilities. Journalized documentations filled office file-cabinets, Internet websites, and universities as students and professors work and study to maintain quality care.
- In the 21st century, I find myself as other individuals, growing older; being filled with knowledge, from reports informing me and the public of improvements. Not merely in technological equipment, research laboratory experience comparisons, or data regarding how or whom should be cited in a negative or positive way.

I want to be informed by media, as how many decreased per capita can be expected to receive humane-care. Statistically speaking, much higher a percent than that of previous era and centuries. It is a concern of mine to tour local facilities, as a visitor, and gather data from research within the sites.

Many hospitals and university medical centers continue to place a good foot forward during inspection times. How many facilities provide adequate to extremely good to excellent care, on a daily, recurring basis? To find such answers it would be impossible by one or two teams of investigators; connecting to the Internet and conveying personal observations, either anonymously or with proper identification, may bring excellence to all facilities. Because that old adage supply and demand will dominate both educational and medical care facilities, no matter how limited the patient load is to the vast array of a metropolitan facility, which cares for both in and outpatients 24 hours a day, 7 days a week, with a non-stop never closing schedule.

Keeping in mind that not all patients require or need equal treatment, in terms of major or minor surgery; often, special allocations are arranged for intensely long-term nurturing for a variety of purposes. For instance: *amputees, reconstructive surgical procedural transplants and skin grafts to victims scarred by explosions, accidents, and fire*; these are not pretty sights. Charred bodies with body extremities removed, just not a pretty sight at all. But, things occur that require care. Alcohol or drug addicted newborns, birth defeat babies, and numerous other physical and mental illnesses to patients create problematic concerns for facility care-personnel. Some patients maintain anger beyond lessons and counseling in classroom or by analyst, nurses, and prescription medications. Crippled and handicapped are discriminated enough in the external world, yet, they too are mistreated or over taxed physically to retrain and except their body and mind. Daily discriminations built over the years, of patients' life. After many years of suffering inwardly, often silently, there can rarely be a time when a disfigured man or woman with or without prosthetic devices can be expected to have full-mental faculty; yet, there are many with brilliant minds. Numerous geniuses have contributed not only their physical research to the professionals treating them. Many have contributed the supply and demand for uniquely designed apparatuses for others to benefit from as well. Utilizing all physical and mental awareness can be the only salvation many patients, recovering from injured, remaining under supervision of primary care professionals, require more understanding than one might chose to believe. Mishmoshed bodies can say everything and never speak a work. I know, my face is scarred, my hand is scarred, and various areas on my body have had skin removed to repair me.

How do I feel when someone assumes poor thing? I kind of think how sad individuals believe scars on the outside deplete the internal functions; thinking, reading, researching, and comparing not to mention, accomplish several degrees in a private college. How sad for ignorant and beautiful surface people! Yet, I comprehend their doubts. I too view handicapped or disabled as questionable in regard to their ability or skills at times! Yet tax dollars and private contributions are paid, for such discriminations to be decreased; so disabled individuals can function in an occupation or profession, with reduced snickering.

It seems understanding patients is one task many individuals disregard during research, investigations, and comparisons to the treatment and care over-all in facilities. There is clergy and laypersons within community religious sectors that visit patrons, confined; they would make the best, and probably suspected investigators. They sincere beliefs that all individuals included atheists, Unitarians, non-denominational's, Protestants, Jews, and Catholics alike are under the influence of not a blue sky but that of one god. Therefore, the only prejudicial influences conveyed or portrayed during their religious attributes to patrons, of sector worshipping house would bring their affluence to nurses and patients and all personnel they come in contact.

Me, I care little for "***cover thine ass***" otherwise I would have chosen a fictitious name, to convey this book publicly. My life has been hell; this book can in no-way create its worsening. I lived be five decades (plus a few years) without dying from voicing my opinions. Several instructors, professionals, and neighbors may have wished I dropped dead; at times, the thoughts were mutual. I however get over shit like that because it makes no sense to rehash miserable thoughts or ideas or actions, for longer than it takes to forget the whole thing. My life shall continue I believe beyond old-age about 90; hopefully, not much longer than that! *I'd hate to convey at 91 I need a bedpan and clean linens, to find a grumpy nurse laughing in my face, as I have seen during my youth. That would certainly irk m- big-time!*

Back to reality, visiting merely creates and removes the void, patients bring into a medical emergency room or doctor's office. You know the routine implications I am describing. Nobody cares about the one in room ## so why should we ... type of attitude that follows suit in not only hospitals, universities, charitable organizations, and societies. Its precedence of "why bother" attitudes that destroy otherwise good facilities, and leave patients yearning to be removed to a distant place. Often, negative attitudes provide the onset for <u>negligence's leading to major damages both physically and psychologically</u>, to the particular patients as well as others, observing such on-goings. These following two analogies, in boldface and italics - may clearly convey: ***<u>ignorance is / is not bliss</u>***, as being a most appropriate title for this book; too bad it did not come to mind earlier when I began typing chapters ago!?!

"Blind individuals can see more than we think or believe": they observe via functioning sensory perceptions, conditions and atmospheres as well as ambiance.

- A blind person smells fragrant cologne, hair spray or other odor and scents. The blind person also hears with a more distinct audio-system than we that have all our instincts. Many hear the softest movement because it seems to move the air, in a particular location, as a soft breeze on a hot day.

- Blind individuals as all others with a loss of one or more senses, gain by a self-imposed fear they live with but have come to adjust to – at the onset or after of their loss; developing instincts to a uniquely enhanced level of awareness bring their capacity to deal with darkness, as a playwright or painter creates a beautiful but difficult scene.

"So-and-so has a memory like an elephant": animals recognize human body scents; remembering or retaining the scent indefinitely.

• Ten years or more between to visits to a friend, I wore the same cologne as previously worn; a vicious and treacherous German shepherd dog that my friend brought in from the wintry cold nights in New York, barked for only a few minutes. I stood still for a little while and permitted the dog to observe me. It sniffed my purse, shoes, and attire. I reached down to pat its head or rub its fur, and the animal was completely calmed. Everywhere I went in my friend's house the dog tagged along. When I sat on the sofa, it jumped up and became quite comfortable next to me. That incident gave me a minor role-play of reality. At first I was intimidated and wanted to leave; however, the cologne must have been in the dog's memory. I had not been wearing any clothing or carrying anything the dog would have known. Therefore, that was my observation beginning, on a private but not disclosed level.

• Observing a kitten that I did not want but kept when it was dropped off outside my house, I noticed she didn't like certain guests visiting; not immediately upon their visit. Over a period of time, perhaps a few visits and throughout the weeks as the kitten grew. The kitten ran upstairs as though a vacuum cleaner other loud noise had sounded an alert, instinctually to escape personal damage. She sped away, out of sight till the coast was clear of what might have been harmful. She did not snuggle close to me nor those she one trusted. At first, I though how strange. Then, realizing my kitten was as intelligent as I, filled with instinctual insights actually she was more aware of things than many humans. Individuals do not have a full understand or knowledge of *their* fear-factor; scientifically, experimental projects can be arranged to simulate instances when fear is most prominent. Colleagues and professors not only create simulations, these findings become research documentations, to be used for similar projects as both comparison and evaluation, to decrease the maladjustment.

The one saying or thought from strangers may have an impact upon the society, community, and educational facilities but if negative facts are not clearly defined, no action occurs. Like the blind or ignorant, we all have a tendency to pick and choose which bears value, to us alone.

While working in a medical facility, a frail-elderly patient mentioned the patient in the same room was a pain in the neck; loud annoying always calling out for help in the middle of the night, preventing a good rest. She was correct in complaining. Nurses could not by law issue medications to sedate such a person. A doctor was not listed on the chart! There was a blank-wall for the nursing staff. That to me is neglect, as well as ignoring patients with senility or aggravating disturbances.

Somebody put the patient there. There had to be a doctor's report somewhere, yet, nothing or nobody had answers; that occurred frequently in long-term care facilities. It cannot factually be reported, because to whom would the report for prescriptions be directed? Who would respond with a professional solution? Where would blame be placed or directed if the patient had been taken more ill (as a result of improper administration of sleeping medications); and in fact, would there be any value to the treatment, had someone selected to be in charge If there is no attending, physician, no relative, not one legal loophole to protect facility's and the reputation conveyed by negative or adverse conditions, the public insult, slander and media blasting continues to battle between right and wrong proceeds. Situations arise frequently requiring professional input, immediate response, and monitoring to protect both patient and facility. [Having no authority at all to increase proper sleeping, or care that too me is neglect, once again.]

Such happens in many hospitals, nursing, convalescent home, and hospices. In many jobs, employees neglecting to perform correctly are reprimanded. Employers can terminate those failing to perform. But by the same token, **who is responsible when nobody can be contacted?** Improper acceptance to medical facilities, by unauthorized people, creates many hours of visible and audio unnecessary disturbances. Signatures often cannot be read, do to sloppy handwriting. And, although *who did what to whom should not* be the primary concern; preventing patient well-being injures other patients.

Honestly, reduced staff at nighttime shifts creates more stress on the personnel because it seemed to me, many patients required ambulation to the lavatory, but had to wait long periods of time, sometimes, they were totally ignored as pests. Patients being tested for radiology views, blood workups, and other laboratory related prescribed tests were awakened before the sun shone. They were rarely asked if they needed to go to the rest rooms first, or whether or not they understood the tests ordered, or by whom. I believe silence from professionals constitutes as much negligence as nurses ignoring patients.

Frankly, my observations and previous experience (as a young patient) displayed clear signs that *"patients were treated as last week's trash?"* If you're thinking I'm confused, understand that when you ask a doctor or physician (or any professional in the medical field) *"What's wrong with me?"* That's the first mistake you could make. Conveying statements such as, *"I feel as if I were hit by a truck or just out-of-sorts!"* Another no, no! Patients are aware they aren't dying. Sometimes the fly gets you thinking strangely, incoherent or perplexed. A sincere, understanding response is worth the hour in a doctor's office, the $50.00 or more office visit cost, and perhaps even that expensive prescription; but when insincerity reeks its time to seek out different medical care-providers.

"You're alive. You may live for thirty or more years." or *You could also die when you cross the street, by a moving vehicle."* Often the preceding statements can be heard as jestfully and non-conclusive. Maybe I exaggerate but doctors get asked *"...am I gonna live through the night?"* Truthfully, how can a doctor reply honestly; he or she is only human and capable of diagnosing the facts. Yet, many doctors and patients fail to

review logical inferences, during critic moments. Keep in mind by the physician is truly accepted as a professionally qualified healer, the training has been in depth throughout the doctor's adult life. Many doctors have practiced some many years, they too require physician's care but refuse to accept the inevitable natural aging process. The older the doctor - or the nurse for that matter, the more reflective look backs into that youthful acceptance and Hippocratic Oath and all the requirements become brought into focus. It appears young doctors and elderly doctors stress the importance of professional guidelines. Those in practice for more than five but not beyond their retiring years seem to betray their professional undertakings; not all, but a small percentage.

Detecting negligence and reporting it leave our hearts in a shamble and individuals just aren't what they used to be, because politicians and other admired or respected leadership groups often focus upon a specific topic, subject, or condition. One way to bring neglect out in the open might be to simply ask for assistance, by an employee during a visit, to a loved-one. Make a mental notation of the response – verbal and body language portrayed. Jot down the number of times you hear or see a light outside other patient's rooms; flickering or beeping usually conveys someone needs or wants help. Rooms with intercoms have greatly reduced that frivolous walk for the nursing staff, from desk to patient rooms. However, how long did it take for an actual reply from the desk, can save a life or contribute to the harm or even death? And before you leave from your visit, ask yourself, "*Would I come to this place for care when sick?*"

That basic question not only removes fear, if your answer is yes; it conveys your best opinion. Oh, before you get too happy with the beauty and hominess of the staff, observe odors as you pass patient rooms en route to the elevator or other exit. "*Do you smell urine? Feces…? Soured milk or other signs of stale food products, possibly growing fungus?*" There are only a few ways to detect that which is normally, undetectable. A guileful way to inquire is directly **ask**, for a cup of coffee or tea (for: yourself). **Observe** [again] responses you receive (from: a nurse, aide, housekeeper or dietary assistant); **create** an additional mental notation. If you receive a cup of coffee or an explanation of sort, don't be afraid to remember it. **Jot down,** *"whether you were issued it with creamer packets or liquid milk, sweetener or sugar, and its temperature. Was it scolding hot or drinkable?"* Now here's the tricky part; you have to be honest.

"Did the person bring you coffee return to check who was drinking it?" This too is a way of learning about regulations, by staff in a facility. If the patient is on a strict diet, you should be informed not to drink or share it with that person. A nurse should request you drink it in the waiting room or at the nurses' station, to avoid the patient from asking for a sip. However, if you are refused, and it is a reasonable time of day or evening- this could represent that you are becoming a bother. *"If your pal, mom, dad, or loved one is being cared-for in a facility, their bill could surely afford a twenty five cent cup of coffee or tea; don't you think?"* I was once fired from a job for issuing a beverage to a visitor. How strange!?! How downright strange!

I know many medical professionals care; many are wonderful. I am not including every medical professional when I create a minor scenario for detecting neglect. My intent is to alert individuals before they are patients, before complaints, questions are left piled on a desk or in a folder of a cabinet nobody opens. As horrendous as politics are without a conveyance of complaints and praises, leaderships and community groups or committees would not be necessary. In a perfect world, there is no need to convey or pass judgment. In the real world, without input no changes or corrections can ever become redefined, evaluated, tested, and improved. Keep in mind that facilities are not merely properties of one individual, with greedy intentions; there are corporations, insurance companies, and government owned establishments. Private sectors assume there facility is unapproachable by government because there are no taxed dollars contributing to the care or treatment of its patients. The more I edit and revise the original book's context, I realize must indeed report its profits and losses to the governing powers, such as shareholders, stockholders, and the federal government for which it submits annual income and expense reports (for the purpose of monthly and quarterly contributions by both the facility and employees). Therefore: private institutions, schools, colleges, universities, emergency and/or long-term medical facilities each must answer to the financial donor. Applying for government funds in the of a loan, grant or equipment development or modernized technological machinery grants access as well, for public information to be aired by investigative news-reporters.

As of the 1970s many filings grant historic and current-day reference, to investigative and private individuals. Comparisons of one inquiry to another and a combination of all, can be disclosed or reported, by anyone, supposedly without fear of slanderous legal-action being brought against the horn-blower; I should know, but that's not the way society works! Angry owners and loved-ones continue to battle the end-result, leaving numerous questions unanswered. Reference according *'the right to know,'* policy for the disclosure act's creation, defined the way in which I, you, and just about anyone with Internet access is availed references; frequently, anonymously or via one's true identity. We need not leave our homes, purchase periodicals and newspapers, nor do we truly require collaboration with colleagues or employers, to received background checks on private citizens or facilities. Public interest became focused on available data through years of combative malpractice allegations. Widening the horizon, inquiries to everyone including the competitors, in occupational, educational, privately owned & operated facilities globally; not stopping there, personally data can be dug-up within minutes to a few hours, of employees, professors, leaders, politicians, neighbors, relatives, or whomever. Somehow, references remain, unexposed or overly exploited. *"Why?"*

Somewhere, I was told that a private, medical facility, did not have to comply with government standards; but, even when the facility does not apply or receive any government funds, to provide adequate patient care or facility structure, a major dispute is clear. Medicare does provide a majority funds for elderly, in long-term facilities; it supplies funds for prescription medications, syringes, proper storage of equipment and electronic patient machines, beds, wheelchairs, the in annual tax forms, all facilities file income and output of funds. Benefits are issued according to the annual reports and funds than are either decreased or increased, as the facilities grow or linger, professionally. Big businesses do not concern the daily dollar for dollar rationale' as home-owners and entrepreneurs do. **Big business** leaders seek tax-free funds and contributions untraceable. Financial payments, furthermore by the indirect means of the (American) government override all the privacy laws, for businesses. **Medicare** was set-up to protect those that had contributed; it was not inclusive of the wealthy, indigent, nor did it set along boundaries of the mediocre 'middle-class'. My researched references, in a chapter ahead, open the funding policy of facilities a little further; including where and how many Medicare funds can be provider within a select professional-office or facility, for specific patient-types of care.

Alternate *private sector care*, which can become available is nice if facilities receiving patient funds are independent of *government tax-breaks* and/or direct Medicare contributions from Social Security. Employees injured on the job, frequently have been accused of abusing funds, allocated specifically by employers, in the form of contributions to: "**Worker's Compensation.**" The government affiliated agency **Worker's Compensation** created to protect corporations from individual lawsuits that could financial destroy businesses, is governed by financial taxation of employers. Each employer (corporate or private) must disclose wages earned by employees as well as contribute to the "**WC**" fund. There are no company or corporations nor private employers free of this contribution; it is maintained for the protection of big businesses as well as the care for injured employees and their families, during a time when physical (and possibly job-related psychological) injuries prevents continued employment.

At times, I think *donating personal and professional information to agencies is crude and uncalled-for*. Disclosures of any kind, have a way of backfiring; my husband believe, "S*ay nothing; never volunteer information.*" He, I have come to believe, is often smarter than most people. Disclosures from terminated or potentially terminated employees proved to be a hoax, as some submit fake *on-the-job injuries;* which pass generalized review, create the sailing-along life's path, collecting funds illegally. They display no concern, for those truly injured in-need. Yet, the reality to such on-goings occur in every region at one time or another, unchallenged; the results, depleted funds by disgusted and those refusing to contribute to a scam-like agency!

The statements above may appear as fickle, harsh, and infantile. Frankly each does in-effect create a *major-concern* for graduates, en route to business success. Barriers however, undetectable fraud, and handled prominent ***"Mission Statements"*** in presentations to the public and fundraisers, assisting daily business. In knowing anyone can claim to be injured and entitled to compensation, before many aspiring business leaders begin, they are faced with in-calculative and potential devious employees; failing to screen and employ honest individuals has no place in the arena of professionalism. As distasteful as "*government image has become,*" stricter enforcement is necessary; only – "*to whom???*"

"*Where is the sense to it?*" and "*How can **fact from fiction** be ascertained true without prolonging the collection process, by proper claimants?*" The Social Security Administration, the Internal Revenue Service, and the big-brother-syndromic fallacy (often believe to be phony) continues auditing and observing employee and employer activities. Here in the these United States however wonderful freedom is noted-as being, there are facets which create delusions, unattainable heights; failures created not by ignorance in accounting or estimating specific contractual work. More often it is failure because of that free-enterprise imagery, new businesses envision, leaving themselves and their businesses, fully unprotected. If I am misrepresenting facts, then perhaps I did not absorb as much in the Accounting II course, as I was supposed-to during that horrendously intimidating and mentally taxing study in 2001 & 2002.

A small-percent of the public believes attorneys and judges have abundant knowledge, in business and legal matters. Anyone completing high school, continuing educational pursuits or seeking a *two or four year*, degree in a university, has equal if not more capabilities. Their qualifications to not only pursue future standards but to question errors surfacing slowly, trickling deeply in pockets of laypersons through economic falsehoods. The individuals create demands, for services, as modern inferences readily focused upon improvements. *Graduates* possess compelling advisory skills, and proficiency in diverse businesses that often requires embellishment, by: <u>seminars, conferences, and the voiced opinions</u>, evaluating consumer's needs as the priority.

Portraying a dedication to advance professionally, keeping current with modernized business develops investigators of tomorrow. It has been proven repeatedly in a wide spectrum that individuals networking locally, tend to remain there. Networking globally at seminars online, in universities, or private conferences conveys professionalism to a consumer, customer, client relationship, as well as enhancing knowledge. Oration of personal observations in multiple locations provides comparable visual; each visual presents positive and negative economic growth and development. The medical facilities with limited funding, extreme debt, and carry over vacant patient rosters deplete economically the power of professional services. Overly crowded medical facilities have become the starting point within 'government assisted' facilities; many of which have been forewarned by economists, students, and accountants. However, much of the observations more often than not do not provide solutions, for accessibility, of payments.

This process though long and dragged out, of observing and reporting, deplete what has not been accomplished; it may however redevelop into a factual-notation, to be stored away, for business and possibly, personal reference to form a regime that increases patient care and treatment, facility maintenance, and personnel salaries. Overhead costs also portray a strong venue of economic failures, to facilities, which have been periodically subsidized by government funding. Government subsidies do not last forever; therefore administration must conquer the failure to abide by 'staying within the means of funds available' to prevent additional overspending frivolously.

Many seminars and conferences are costly. However, facilities are opening their doors to strangers; many of whom, can and will detect all those negative forces, creating determinations of whether or not you, me, or a loved-one would promoted in a good way. Investigative reporters do not merely seek one area of professional inquiry. One area is not under assault. It is the entire cycle to business related functions, which become affected by neglect. I cannot stop it alone. I cannot prove it alone. I alone cannot truly be at more than one location at a time without casting hostile removal. Keeping my petty but factual mind-teasers close at hand; visiting a sick person can become the beginning of a new, well needed, career for the inquisitive mind.

Closing this chapter with a saddening event, in the late 1990s, I have been led down a path of destroyed hope, in a couple of medical facilities. Personal observations, complaining to management, and jotting memos brought no changes; it was unnoticed, as its leadership cast patients aside. Families not out of lack of concern for the safety and well-being opted to provide homecare. The patients too ill for homecare continued their stay in medical facilities, lacking sufficient staff and treatment, as economically depleted funds just fumphered.

- *1980s A relative was diagnosed with* **H.I.V./A.I.D.S.** *I had not become alert to the illness during previous studies, in the course of <u>geriatric health</u>; yet, the diagnosis was not new to my ears, to others. I had heard-of it during my childhood, as a patient, being cared-for during the 1950s. God knows it was so long ago maybe I was three or four years old. I possessed a minimal understanding of the illness; rationalizing it as <u>simple garb!</u>*

- *My knowledge included little to sooth my psychological gut-feeling; I would be loosing my brother, at one time. To make matters worse, one of my adolescents also was diagnosed; he too contracted the disease. I, - a caring and medically-concerned individual - desired improvements for all patients, faced with such difficult facts. The illness was a disease I could not or perhaps, did not wish to face nor believe could have truly latched-on to anyone in my family.*

- *I found my minimal-knowledge challenged by beliefs, filled with thoughts and questions, such as: "It was a sexual-related illness."*

- *"My brother was a mere youth; he lived only within a year of his twenty-first birthday; suffering for a few years, once his diagnosis turned to a negative-prognosis."*

- *"My son was married; he worked toward my beliefs, for family-continuity of a lifestyle I had been led to believe was essential, for a happy home. His suffering lingered once his diagnosis had been confirmed, for nearly a decade. His widow and son emotionally scarred; will they survive? Will any survivors truly encourage diagnostic examinations? Why must unnecessary examinations be scheduled as early-detection - as the determinant - for human-beings to: <u>sleep better at night, enjoy 'greater' sexual-gratification, and develop communities based upon mode-family-images portraying falsehoods that continue to outnumber honesty taught in many sectors, as religion condescends?</u>*

- *My sister and I, we have a mother that has not ever been up to intellectual acceptable standards throughout our lifetimes.* *We {more so my sister than I} contributed emotional support, so our mother could succumb to her future with dignity.*

    1. ***"How, many other families face the anger, I have described briefly?"*** ***"How many more familiar faces grow thin, with frail bodies before their natural aging-process begins?"***

    2. ***"And why young, potentially decent human-beings diagnosed with horrendously, emotionally crippling diseases, project hazardous encountered, for the naïve public?"***

- *All the why, how, what for-s cannot reduce my emotional burden nor those of others, as we each cope with dilemmas of personal growth and development, en route to the future. Somewhere there are answers. Somehow there will be cures. Sometimes, I wish it were I that had been diagnosed; knowing I'm a big coward, I would most likely fight to my death, as I fight arrogance and neglect in my life.*

- *"What the hell good is anything I convey or do; I could not detect illness in its early stage, to create the desired reversible diagnoses, saving those two special individuals?"*

- *Numerous scientific experimentations relayed message to the public and private sector, of disease contracted via blood-transfused, mucous-transferred, and such terminological words, frequently meaning nothing to me and others till it actually hit home (as they say). HIV/AIDS once introduced to the public, led newspapers headlines and broadcast bulletins alarming people. The conveyance of cause-and-effects of the disease created near panic. Fear of becoming involved with a sick-person; one infected, ready to attack unsuspecting individuals followed. Near plague-like mentalities swarmed to private physicians as well as public healthcare centers, to be tested. The wonderful 1980s became my dilemma; tossing away medical cares, I canceled my thinking for fear that I would be next. What would happen to my spouse, adolescents still alive and well, and how my future will be as the void that nasty gut feeling of emptiness, build my emotions back to a decent level, for basic existence. such thoughts and fears covered my days and nights. How often I'd find myself in a simple conversation, tears flowing, as though I were in unbearable physical pain? This chapter has taken its toll on my ancestry, in a small facet of living, but I shall continue to pursue whatever changes and complaints being brought forth, in a hope the public will not become victims any longer – to a silent undetectable neglect.*

- *Confusion, anger, and misunderstanding took place. An inner dispute: wanting to believe those two diagnoses were untrue, yearned to hear, "April fool's!" My comfort was not found. I pursue, periodically attending and visiting the infirmed, in a hope to conduct a better comparison for all emotional views, to alleviate what I still will not be capable of changing.*

- *The **HIV/AIDS** virus had grips on young, aspiring, and wonderful people; the elderly became frail, and required home-health-care. Hundreds of diseases flood the* Taber's Cyclopedic Medical Dictionary *that I own and read, from time-to-time, for personal knowledge and during educational 'geriatric healthcare' course. There are no guarantees diagnostics are accurate, for all patients. A cures for one individual as a remedy cannot factually be documented, as becoming accurate for **all patients;** . therefore, I truly believe the obligation of all individuals is to secure a method of concern. Forming an factual way to set guidelines, in identifying illnesses. This may not be the answers for all dilemmas but it provides accurate revelations required by the medical industry, to either develop or properly treat illnesses with cures proven to be effective.*

- *As with any medical problem, the public does not possess a mastering to identify an ailment just as many business topics, of deep concern require professional decisions nobody should live with the question I have, for many years! "Oh, they'll think I'm an idiot?"*

Better you are thought to be idiot today than you are proven idiotic in the future. Then it's too late. As my brother and my son both died from incurable-diseased bodies, they might have been healed with logical thinking, instead of **"that can't be we're family; you can't be sick!"**

A zillions questions and orations conclude the most important truth, for me and many others blurting at me by my daughter, momentarily created an air of hate; she seems judgmental to my feelings of wishful thinking "*Mom, you're in denial*!" I could not face those facts. Such attitudes enhance diseases and remove all possible hope for cures.

This chapter was a blessing to research. Okay, not right away!

Delving into ***dictionaries, encyclopedias, periodicals, and researching references in public libraries***, for input, interesting to the public and finding data overwhelmed me; I printed 'this-and-copied-that' till I decided to create a file on my computer. It was intriguing. I, an intelligent woman, creating my own criteria collection; one technological facet of this research let to another. Not wishing to print out numerous pages to rummage through at home, I decided to transmit the researched data, to myself. Trust-me it did not seem possible. As overwhelming and mind-boggling as that seems, it was a breeze! A very time-consuming breeze! The barricades early-on became minor dilemmas, in complete control by a technology-system I once feared. Not because I was computer illiterate. My fear was if I can access vast and complex research projects independently as a novice, more or less where does technology draw the line?

My research criteria or technique or style of queries occasionally demanded a rephrasing query. As I began implementing my professionally learned format, valhol, an entire world opened. Flooded by this newfound brilliance, I confronted other challenges from my house, for book-length references.

Seeking answers by: *acquaintances, associates, and professors at college* inferences were minimal; colleagues rarely contribute anything, freely. Somehow, I found myself beginning to believe references, of antecedence was curtailed, for investigative reporters of prominent television and radio broadcasting stations. My continued search, along with my neighbor's daughter via the Internet, at local libraries and from within my house, our two minds focused in unison. Talking out the process to accurately achieve, more detail than I would have believed available. The data I have included in this book's section does not reflect further back than the 1880s.

According to the ***Britannica Encyclopedia*** in 1847, there were 250 delegates within the **A**merican **M**edical **A**ssociation [**AMA**]. They gathered and combined their wisdom to create and setup several **M**edical **H**ealth **C**enters. The first one of great recognition was established during 1910; its home was Wilkes Barre, Pennsylvania. It was the path for many communities to follow, to give access locally to patients, in need of care, and to utilize community facilities, for preventive ailments.

These centers brought the need for nurses to be professional. In 1919 the **N**urses **A**ct established the **G**eneral **N**ursing **C**ouncil, for England and Wales, to maintain a register of nurses. Similar acts were passed in Scotland, at the times, as well. In the years to follow Northern Ireland entered into the agreement, in 1922. As the field of registrants grew in Europe and around the world, so did the need for a new council. In 1946 the **N**ational **H**ealth **S**ervice had the say in an act accepted in 1949; it consolidated all previous acts and established regional committees, to work in schools of nursing.

The **W**orld **H**ealth **O**rganization included nursing in its activities, from its beginning, in 1948. Member nations requested assistance in developing educational programs, for: *nurses, auxiliaries and midwives, and to organize public health programs and hospitals*. Countries are assisted in establishing nursing, as part of the *national health departments*. Governments aided in the establishment of *nursing and nursing-education systems*, also. **WHO** (World Health Organization) discovered in many countries more than half of all the births are attended by untrained midwives. ***Fellowships*** granted to nurses, for overseas study when consultants from the ***WHO*** worked in the countries; they strive to leave *national counterpart personnel*, to continue their work. Study outside the country (the USA and foreign lands) may be needed to develop such personnel.

In 1979 according to the Britannica Encyclopedia's reference a **C**entral **C**ouncil, for **N**ursing**, M**idwifery, and **H**ealth **V**isiting has national boards, for the four parts of the United Kingdom. It became responsible for instruction, registration, disciplinary machinery, and all post basic-education (including *health visiting, district, and school nursing)*.

On paper or computer disks, recorded data appears to be fabulous, for patients. Data states nursing students continue, in affiliated sectors, to pursue careers as do-gooders. The data available brings out the best of a profession that has been advancing, from the

19th and 20th centuries. It does not include historic datum regarding medical ethics; *torts* filed by irate patients attorneys were not included.

Criminal assaults believed to have occurred, by physicians, especially to emotionally ill patients, and much of the historic data excludes their pharmaceutical needs often frowned upon, by many individuals in good health, calling for a new cure-all drug, to be developed and administered. Available data shows **responsibility within the medical profession** not only includes nurses, giving treatment to the injured, ordered by physicians but all persons, to prevent harmful situations from occurring. It is the responsibility of employees to not only prevent patient injury; it is a required obligation to avoid casting irresponsible activities, in the work place, which could lead patients doubting the physician's or staff's qualifications. Monitoring employees is not often considered an obligation of co-workers; but, it is!

Think about this: *millions of dollars are issued in settlements* by courts of law, to criminals, who claim malpractice from their physician(s). Those dollars deplete medical facilities, laboratories, and associated/private practices of physicians striving to meet quantitative employee/er rosters, for a smooth efficient practice. States maintain Licensing Boards require Educational Standards for Registrants, in most professions. *Physicians* and *Nurses* are no different. They must pass examinations <u>even</u> *after graduating* their school of training. Photo Identification, Fingerprinting, Application, and Annual Fees are the start of a future, for those qualified with a desire to be in a field of medicine. After years of working in the same atmosphere, some jobs become a ritualistic dilemma. Physician, nurse, aide, dietary worker, and just about all others in many jobs find humdrum-like side-affects. There is a rare fellow employee acquaintance, to discuss shunned feelings or self-defeat, of being a successful person in a world of illness, dying, births, and emergency care centers. That point reaches different individuals at various times; timing has little to do with deeply embedded harm lived by patients, desiring to get well.

Throughout my life I have wondered and hoped for a better world; especially, in the medical aspect of living. It has yet to be viewed {by me} even though there are remarkable changes for the better, in globalized care and treatments to patients. In the 1970s while working Private Duty as a Home Health Aide, for the elderly, handicapped, or whomever I was assigned by an agency I found *individuals thought quite the same. **Furthermore, many were dissuaded of thoughts about being incorrectly being charged on billing statements, from doctors or facilities, for treatments.*** Those patients were being financially burdened, at costs to insurance companies and government funding.

Facts: A patient with private medical insurance (or ***cash payments***) rarely has somebody to turn to for assistance or guidance, regarding billing errors. Patients being treated that have Medicaid are treated much to my surprise, as if they were derelicts. Not because they were; because society dictates such abuse. When a country or city health department closes, emergency rooms, according to laws in various states, are supposed to and expected to treat all patients. However, private facilities do not have to comply with such expectations. **Why…?** If you read the previous chapter much of the funding-grants are received from government loans; which are far less repayment interest rated than banks or personal lenders. Medicare patients *many of whom have provided a percent of their salaries for twenty, thirty, or many, many more years* have found, they are being denied [**proper**] *sufficient treatment, laboratory testing, quality care by a physician* (of their choice) *and they are responsible for at least 20% of **all** billing*, for: ***accepted ailments, tests, prescriptions, office visits, etc.*** During the 20th century, Medicare patients also had come to find there are additional costs for, Vision and Dental needs.

Questioning the cost of an ***aspirin*** (or other prescription), ***bedpan*** (usage for bedridden patients, post-op or examination of urine or feces), ***a box of tissues*** and ***goody pack*** (once admitted for observation or treatment to a facility), ***meals*** (they receive as an overnight patient, several days, recuperative time or any addition to other treatments) are discouraged, from furthering inquiries. Especially, the *elderly* or *custodian* responsible, for the costs' they are treated as if they were imagining dual or high-costs for tests, applications of treatments or other care which they are certain was not administered. According to articles written during the 1970s, benefits for _Long-Term Care_ was below average costs. Where?

Therefore, payments should be increased to improve the quality, and care desired. And, during the latter part of the 1980s that **_topic_** was mailed to _Social Security Recipients,_ of spousal or dependent check receivers; the notification to them was that '**_they needed to purchase Extended Medical Insurance_**' to reduce their burdens, in their future. Extended Medical Insurance for many on fixed incomes was the start of one more annoyance; declared a rip-off, by columnists and publicists around the U. S. of A. Many talks were conveyed with Congress and Social Security Administration delving into ways of curtailing increases; however, asking any retired individual how much their Medicare Contributions varied in the 20^{th}C and currently in the 21^{st}C. Reply will be additionally increased from $25.00 to $75.00+ monthly, depending on the assessed contribution against the deductions; and from this rate of monthly deductions, from supposedly Tax-Free income, will increase at the cost of living 2.5+ percent, however only a 1.5% to 5.%, annual increase of fixed incomes monthly will be issued**!**

"**_If that one situation does not make you sick, than you must have plenty of, frivolous money to repay what have been prepaid, many times over!_**" This is merely my personal opinion. Leaderships and administrators, along with numerous colleagues might think I was badmouthing the system. The data in this book compares to personal research as well as facts from not only documented research reports, by the government; reported criteria has references to back up, in the form of periodical and newspaper articles (published weekly/monthly), and the like. I alone do not criticize a system without the strength of far more superiorly educated and occupationally included commentators, of the Wall Street Journal, New York Times, The Miami Herald (and Broward Edition), and the Kipling Newsletter/Report. Much more data referred to is accessible in _public library and resource centers_, in municipalities throughout the USA and over the internet worldwide.

Data is not privately accessible; it is available to the public, in globally explorations, for knowledge. Modern technology has brought countries together and distantly, although far apart in the interests and concerns for its people!

More criteria frequently '***pushed under the rug***' include unemployment. They too find themselves feeling ripped-off, by plans/insurance companies they paid to protect them, during a time of health needs. My background educationally and employment accomplishments, volunteering in my community increased my observationary, individuals interests. Mainly during volunteering for the sake of freeing parents' minds, to work as their adolescents hung around poolside, or in a local playground brought to the surface conditions not negative, rather incapable individuals not providing aging parents' care.

I have seen them (the aging parents, grandparents, etc.) when they felt great, miserable, and curious with concerns for loved ones during a medical crisis. They react pretty much as I, pondering what can be done to ease symptoms of pain, stress, and how can healing being smoothly coerced. Devastated by long waited in emergency rooms designed to create ample care, in a crisis. Critical thinking delves silently at times: "***Where are those agencies which are well-known for their contributions in fields of community health centers when individuals are lingering, in pain, on gurneys?***" I am still asking simple, unanswerable questions, by more superior or intelligent beings than I. Genuine concern can create changes; however, there is more than one element that requires meeting advancements. It is necessary for improvements, to provide affordable, and decent care. Research I seek in library archives, past and most recent articles in periodicals, provide butterflies, as I refill my desk with notations, papers jotted with queries, and the original version of this book. The book written rapidly, during a college break between degrees. I wanted to create a book with agility to transform, from a derogatory fact-statement into a blossoming, peace-of-mind piece of work. Frowns are remaining, as I continue to read, observe, and research data, referring to newly formed agencies and associations, to help people, to help individuals improve their lives for the future.

Surmised unspoken opinions include queries regarding <u>Associations, Councils, and Legal Acts</u>. Many unworthy of *ethical activity; a*pparently, it cannot stop. Doctors, nurses, and other medical facility personnel are required to maintain a trail of paperwork. Reports are passed to organizations, findings of conditions and treatments, and useful input for care or prevention of diseases. Documenting is a leader in bypassing patient care for positive as well as negative results. Documentation required by governments, insurance actuaries, statistics for organizations in regional centers as comparisons are necessary, to adjust valuable dollars to maintain sufficient care. Anticipated needs and outcomes of surgical experimentations are reported, for advancement or breakthroughs, in a specific field of study, to compare with worldwide studies. Numerous clusters of paperwork, technology files, and seminar oration open doors to the public and professionals, all seeking a better way.

Improvements with volunteers, employees hired to sort through abundant data make valuable input the asset necessary when properly maintained and reported. Preparation does not deplete life-sustaining care; it is a foundation not for the formation of governing departments, agencies, and associations. **Preparation** should be the primary function for any physician, nurse, and related care giving personnel. In the long run medical costs will not decrease with riveting knowledge; it is my belief that the entire medical cost will become less burdensome. Patients' households, elderly and/or Medicare and Medicaid patients, and professionals will gain respect, for the paying the price of honestly and genuine customer care.

As global reports continue to become accessible publicly, in regard to malpractice, it creates a doomed feeling to the potential patient. A reflection of the lack of governing, by organizations that claim to desire putting an end to negligence. Reports from organized-medical groups, and patients often believe their lives will be an asset, as '***big-brother-syndromic***' focuses secretly as *watch over-ers. Professional, family, volunteers* or *friends* were judged not by ***knowledge, ability, skill*** or their available ***awareness*** *for both previous and modern times.* Many individuals are judged by the projected concern for a patient. Observing damage, others claimed to receive or heard to have been issued gave professional care individuals, a bad name. Committees of physicians, nurses, attorneys, and lay individuals were formed *to hear and decide outcomes,* for legal actions. The procedure opened doors to ***money***, to a person with a good attorney, if there was a good amount at the end of the rainbow, to be gained by falsely accusing a care-giver/care-taker. My personal thought remains to sympathize with high judicial award, by private or other means to criminals; when caught are they made to repay the granted settlement back, with interest? Do they go scot-free to enjoy the lap-of-luxury, in non-reciprocal countries; basking in the sun on beautiful beaches or skiing the highest down-slope while the sued professional stands in long lines at the unemployment office, welfare centers, and re-educational facilities because he or she cannot be considered employable or trust-worthy?

> The results of committees proved improper and were criticized within their prospective area-of-expertise. However, ***malpractice*** ran *havoc in the United States of America and globally,* as well for a full decade, non-stop! In the 1960s, a patient could be mistreated, neglected, abused, and possibly wrongfully diagnosed causing severe physical and psychological lasting effects. The incidents, many unreported, were the foundation for inquiries by frightened (for fear of being terminated from the employment and/or being ruined, at the educational pursuit levels toward advancement). With silent sneering and reduced hourly schedules or increased work-shifts, and other persuasive tactics, medical personnel shivered, in view of negligence.

It is a terrible thing to question that which I do not have answers to. It is far more humiliating when governing powers do not have solutions, to recreate that which once developed foundations with good-intentions, to permit antecedence to fumble. I wish I knew or had the ability and capacity to be invoking a better system. I believe I am not quite ready for that deeply, time-consuming chore.

During that clash of opinion, insurance rates in both private and facility offices skyrocketed. There was no foundation standing up for the good guys. No agency cast kindness upon medical personnel without being criticized by aggressive reporters, and attorneys with dollar signs in the eyes. A majority of professional physicians closed their practices. Many grouped together, to afford escalating insurance premium rates, too costly for a single practitioner. Others, mostly more advanced in their years of practicing medicine, they chose to leave their immediate state, for a newfound practice, unscarred by malpractice and high insurance premiums. Moreover, a small handful of professional physicians entered into a brotherhood of secrecy, to remain in private practice, for their trusting patients. Is there any good to hiding behind closed doors, watching a profession denigrated, and nearly destroyed for the financial growth, of liars? Are no noble and reliable sources within many associations, agencies, departments, and organizations to withstand the trials-and-tribulations, facing decent individuals? And, as sad as this may seem, I too have no soothing pun, antidote, and there seem to be nothing substantial for the public, private, and professional sectors to do, to practice any desire occupation – with worries of failure in their path to success. Granted, I did research and access:

State Laws that are being updated as I write.

International Laws adding addendum clauses, limits financial restitution awarded.

Insurance Companies include subrogate clauses, for purchasers.

With laws providing less risk to students, both men and women once being turned away from care related occupations, returning to universities and medical centers, there may be a brighter future as we each approach varying shades of our rainbows.

Conflicts which are never going to be simple or quick to avoid, may increase previously organized foundations, to utilize the newly brought into focus and documented legal adaptations; required to improve that which once was perfect but by the power or greed – had vanished from its caring standing.

The primary cause for the laws to be changed was doctors of the 1980s were forced to pay insurance premiums beyond any reasonable income. It was not escalated to destroy practices. Administrators of medical facilities, increased the entrance-level requirements of new personnel not just physicians and licensed nurses; receptionists, billing and accountant departments, and each housekeeper and maintenance employee was given lessons in CRP and simple First Aid Treatment. This practice was an embarrassment with good outcomes. It focused the employees shift, in a medical facility for what it was; a caring center. Each employee was unofficially obligated to know the life-saving care for an emergency, on the job, to reduce the time required by emergency teams to responds. Although this may seem frivolous, it became the standard for future employment, and it was and I thinks is a good idea to continue, for as long as we expect to be treated properly.

Groups of professions might create questions - *patients are not too happy with but some thoughts are more necessarily considered after a horrendous problem arises* - such as:

- *"Who is / was the doctor?"*
- *"What does the doctor know about treating their ailment, and that of every individual?"*
- *"How many doctors will be available for the patient especially during a crisis or emergency?"*
- *"Do new associated or affiliated doctors have ample knowledge to handle full case loads during, the absence of a team leader* or *assigned physician?"*

Answer came to mind between the 1970s and 1980s; insurance companies proved to be enveloped, in money charged for care and treatments to patients covered, than ever before. No only did insurance companies discontinue an ease in which previously utilizing authority to cancel a patient's coverage for multiple ailments or accidents, subrogation clauses became more actively functioning. Insurance companies began seeking the *"whys"* of many clients? [as numerous similar injuries repeatedly had been submitted for payments]. It was also discovered, third party involvements contributed, to misrepresentation of injuries, as the culprit. The once *doctor-patient-legal system priorities* rose to greater heights, than projected by actuarial analysts and knowledgeable business and financial wizardry. The triage-of-concern, developed into a square. The four sided concern among *insurance companies-doctor-patient-legal system* was born. It offered less time consuming crap, by evaluating incident and accident reports and required treatments found patients and financiers much happier than ever before. The high of insurance, however, did not reduce for medical care tremendously.

With one concern made less stressful came a new crisis for patients and professionals, unpreventable specializations were the norm. Organizations did little to the 'specialist' because there would now be a direct, guilty party to place judgments against, during a malpractice legal action, which, as many readers are aware malpractice seemed t have slipped under rugs of the public view and that of Congress and affiliated organizations. So where do we as prospective patients, professionals, and care facility leaders turn in the future? Again, not one clearly definable foundation has thus far been incorporated to divvy up with "*we'll intermediately, evaluate, and present solutions.*"

Do not loose heart, continue reading, for maybe nothing more than the ability to face the future with insight; this in itself reduces my worry when I become ill. Knowing what to say, do, and where to go is essential. How to detect neglect, financial rip-offs, and the potentially required care might be somewhere in this book of babbling. Just do not go to any emergency room for a common-cold, and expect to be treated with immediate open-arms, as you anticipate a physician's professional opinion, for a tablespoon or two of honey and lemon with a hot cup of tea before sleep. It ain't gonna happen. For that you and me, and anyone foolish enough to require medical input, deserves to be ripped-off. And, as humorous as that might seem; it occurs, all too frequently.

In emergency rooms and care facilities, a posted sign identifies the patient's rights. It influentially indicates the obligation to patients and the commitments, by the attending medical teams. However, if that alone does not get your to inquire before retiring to a gurney, you might read the beginning stages of your favorite novel. Lest you are brought in via EMT or Ambulance services, you are merely another patient; unless you truly are bleeding profusely, gasping for air with every breath, and your financial payments can be practically verified within minutes. It's no joke being sick; it leaves you feeling better after that social worker desk, receptionist desk, and the list of on with individuals deciding whether or not you need their care. No medical organizations, foundations, agencies, and certainly not any associations can or will place your body beyond the doors to your recovery or mass confusion, as you wait. That's not what you needed to find out. It is a fact. Ask your neighbors and acquaintances about their bout to ***live and die***.

New policies included with long overdue improvements, and addendums for administrators. It's so easy to have a staff become relaxed, revert to old ways. In many facilities without a watchdog patient care and personnel backslides occur. There is no legal or ethical obligation, during a <u>general suturing, setting of a fracture</u>, and there is little one can do to improve waiting time of non emergencies. I found that out myself; friends and relatives in my view were on gurneys without being observed, for long periods of time. It irked me. I thought what the hell is going on, there's no emergency treatment, a minor skilled individual might have performed. Billing departments in a slue of price ranges are sent demanding payment, for services received. What about the wasted hours in emergency rooms, on a gurney without professional assessment.

Facilities are technically not incorrect, expecting to be paid for the gurney, lighting, air conditioning that we all breathed as patients; linens, pillows, and the latest Paris-fashion gown must be worth some time wasting. In ain't Hospital gowns are not fashionable as buttock, boobs, and blubber is viewed by lifting an arm, leg, or a stroll to the lavatory. Maybe someone with less of a negative attitude can develop something more appropriate.

It seems with millions of taxpayer contributions from payroll deductions, not only should there be an increase of Medical Centers, Long Term Care Facilities, and Rehabilitation Centers for indigents, drug/alcohol addicts; it seems at times our democratic system is not suitable for humans at all. In North Miami Florida, an area sectioned off by some sort of governing power, for experimental reductions to drug abusers had been formed to help or improve local area. At various times I observed while grocery shopping, washing clothes in a Laundromat, en route to work (frequently intimidated as I walked with no coins for the bus), or actually waiting for a bus I and others were harassed, insulted, chased, and for a wallet or handbag. An abundant population, mostly males and a few females dressed in smudged attire, holey shoes, mussed up hair, and soot.

They were drinking alcoholic beverages in old-fashioned lunch bags; smoking marijuana and cigarettes occurred. I think that's a good thing if you can afford it; at least upholding the 1st Amendment's Freedom of 'this and that' in private houses. If they had funds for beer, legal or illegal cigarettes, how come they were victims of society? The same theory is focused on dead beat moms and dads, as they leave because married/family life has no room in their mind. Well, baby, if the family started with two it should continue the façade, of community acceptance till at least offspring can fend for themselves. Why suck off taxpayers for a year or longer? Why are strangers being forced to accept a society that dedicates itself to family and community with slaps in the face, by unworthy beings?

Should I apologize? No, not at all! I'm not holier than thou. I received welfare periodically; my adolescents were Medicaid recipients, at times. I worked and I went to school; then as I found free time as a parent, I returned to college. Okay, so why can't a majority of individuals care that much about the miserable world we all live in. Why indeed?

Because medical centers cannot enforce rules and regulations, to improve a community anymore than individuals living in it; those brilliantly designed architectural structures, on once barren land, soon to follow is bag and baggage will be the same individuals many of us wish to get away from. Again, no solution; I am setting straight my stupid, maladjusted point of view. I am merely voicing my personal opinion of how the world and my lifestyle compete, for the better things in life instead of just complaining and falling into hell.

Publicly soon this damn book is to be self-published and an ISBN will be assigned. It may not be intelligent in one aspect; however, a long journey to old age has my heart and my head clear of once guilt, for accepting other people's financial assistance. Giving back anytime to a community, as a volunteer makes everything less insulting....

In the 1950s community centers brought hope, for safety in medical surgical techniques; patients trusted physicians, nurses, and their corner pharmacists. Not me, unfortunately, I was angry back then. My face and hand were scarred; individuals pointed their nasty fingers at me and yelled, "*stay away from my child,*" and "*go home; you don't belong here.*" As a mature, educated, professional woman, I still hear or overhear, "*Oh, god, hope she keeps going?!?*" And other such arrogance; whatever! *What's to write nice things about? My folks were poor; struggled to meet monthly expenses. I required surgery. But, why I would not accept, psychological understanding or counseling? No, I didn't get a great elementary education; my desire to absorb tons of knowledge & skill, to function in the "real-world" gave me perseverance, not courage to go on. Stamina came from my dad's guidance.*

In the 1960s beatniks were degraded; by individuals like me, I guess with limited mental functions. John F Kennedy approached numerous public schools, bringing about a well needed physical fitness regime, to Junior High School students and the faculties.

In the 1970s rehabilitated or reformed alcohol and/or drug user abusers were degraded; some were medical professionals, and criminally intended legal actions, by fraudulent, greedy folk. Malpractice legal actions surfaced with millions of dollars destroying professionals. The end result forced many honest professionals to reassess their career choices; often what to be doctors, technicians, or nurses turning their study into law.

In the 1980s troubled cities came to a slow-halt; quality production endorsed good construction, in poverty struck locations. Organizations filled with volunteers gave construction of private dwellings, to individuals that did not shun away from physical labor. And so the builders and dwellers became advocates, for others to respect. For decades that followed this building and dwelling entity encompassed the entire United States – as well as foreign countries, as volunteers teamed with professional graduate students, to improve humanity.

In the 1990s medical malpractice reverted; elderly were diagnosed with Alzheimer's, instead of senility; HIV/AIDS destroyed a portion of the population, wiping out numerous patients as the fight to slow or cure the disease became the focal point in medical fields.

In the year **2000** we had crazy, nutzsy folks, renaming everything from socks to undies, computer mouse pads to dinnerware, and paper books to periodical articles entitled Y2K or something! This new millennium made me a little crazier than I would like to believe. I opened '*readme.txt*' files for Y2K reference. Nonsense was perfected, as nearly 805 of private dwellings owned and operated electronic typewriting machines, printers, and internet access – for business and personal communication, at any time of day or night. And more ingratiating any country and even outer space could be communicated to through satellite technology. If that's the complaint I have to contribute, for beginning a new century then the entire population of the United States of America gotta believe - there's finally a positively wonderful time coming, in the future.

Now, I am getting frightened because *previously* when I made such a very happy statement aloud to myself, something horrible occurred. Let's pretend I did not write:

"how sweet this century is making me feel…."

Funding just another word, for *money*; a trade-off of the value of services or physical work, normally under contract. *However*, a contract to develop a structure of beauty with functions other than glamour is a major commitment. The structure requires architectural designers/builders available during problems. *Furthermore*, as beautified an area becomes structures, financial aspects have skyrocketed. All forms of living species require growth and development; frequently within the limitations of parental or custodial protectors, incomes, competition of peers whimsical spending escalates, to meet the area style. *Although* many households claim to be successful financially, they are equally in debt, and global economies often conveyed by reporters in a variety of news-printed articles and orations – share unbalanced economic failings.

__Money__ comes in numerous forms, such as: *coins, currency, and least understood in modern times the barter-system*. This fundamental creation was developed not only to get what you deserve, for your products or services; the system of denominational-worth perceived during negotiations, for its personal time and efforts. Value of a product or service varies; no two services are truly '*__precisely__*' alike. Just as there are variations in services, products can not '*__all__*' be compared as equally valuable. In *institutions, factories, facilities, and public resource centers*, value of care perceived, by *consumers, clients,* in this particular book *__patients__* that have or have been issued care and treatments, to aid in the healthiness (physical and/or mental state of mind), have proved to be debatable often.

As critical thinking revealed varying balanced levels of facility needs verses patient needs, a slue of queries arose. Costs of patient care, one of the most under estimated aspects might be better off with our monetary system. There is however an antiquated value, from the beginning of time typically, still in use in modern times. This barter system has a few questions and answers from an internet search, which can develop other questions. For the most part of bartering, medical centers and medical professionals do not appear within a realm of adequate use. Insurance companies might benefit by a barter system, as its products supplied to medical facilities, for patients care, could become an effective reduction to the manufacturing of prescription and over the counter medications. Obviously, the balancing act of barter system's usefulness would require meeting a preliminary ratio, of supply and demand. In such a scenario for medications, insurance companies (especially for senior citizens) cut monthly prescription prices; equipment required for a patient to remain home, instead of being a long term care individual has also become the norm, in the past 40 years.

Rather than involve my opinion regarding the scale of payment either bartered or monetary perhaps including the outstanding questions located on Yahoo can indulge curiosity of readers, to reconnect their involvement in escalating costs to facilities, patients, and insurance companies. It is also important to never forget the overhead costs, of not only facilities; professional office physicians, their staff, and the location may not be a barter system projectile, as again, daily to weekly costs have a vast deviation.

{**barter**} Q. *How does a barter system work?*

A: A barter system is an old system, which involves exchanging goods and services for other goods and services. This system works effectively in situations where there is no common measure of value to be used in trade.

- *Equipment (i.e.: technology, beds, kitchen & food, etc.) probably could omit 'insurance companies' from out of pocket $$$ - using the system; professionals and their family members could also benefit. It is the everyday neighbor/visitor and emergency room patient that definitely could not have a bartering power.* (2015, Reddock, L's opinion)

Q. What are the advantages of the barter system?

A: According to The Nest, the main advantage of the barter system is its flexibility, which enables the exchange of one product for another. Bartering also helps save money that may have otherwise been used to travel to a shop to buy an item. In some cases, bartering does not entail exchanging or losing the possession of an item. In such cases, service such as maintenance is exchanged for a good.

A key principle of the barter system is that money is not exchanged between the trading partners. A notable difference between bartering and buying is that in the former method, a partner offers an item he does not need in exchange for a desired item. A clear advantage of this method is saving money. In addition, each party gets the item he wants without spending any money. Although it started in ancient times, bartering is used as a mode of trade even in modern times. For instance, there are many online bartering sites on which individuals advertise their items and list the items for which they are willing to trade their goods.

- *Service (injury assessment, monitoring vital signs, and portable equipment) can be equated by the value of its need. Emergency rooms have far more equipment than required, by every patient daily. Mostly equipment in emergency rooms is to restore life and establish the 'what ailment' created a discomfort; the repairing aspect kicks in upon laboratory results, from different equipment, which denotes seriousness of a patient's health. It does not appear barter-able, life threatening or immediate repair by suturing, bandaging, and medicating. (2015, Reddock, L's opinion)*

Q: Who uses the barter system today?

A: Bartering is a popular form of trade for individuals, families, and businesses seeking to save money. Some small and medium sized businesses join bartering networks to exchange various goods and services. Barter networks help businesses grow by brokering deals to exchange items such as copiers, phone systems, work shirts, carpet cleaning, and even real estate.

Through bartering, a retail business can get rid of excess inventory. Service providers also use bartering to fill an excess capacity of hours. For instance, a dentist who has an extra five hours a week to fill can barter five hours of dental work in exchange for useful goods or services. Some bartering networks provide members with a line of credit, which is then used similarly to a bank loan. For example, a restaurant can barter for construction services to build additional space, instead of seeking a traditional bank loan to fund the project.

Another group that finds bartering helpful is low-income families. Some low-income families form private bartering networks for purposes of exchanging food, car rides, and other essential items. Bartering groups such as the Black Women's Blueprint sustain families through hard economic times. Individuals who wish to get rid of unused items can exchange them for goods and services at websites such as Swap.com.

- Property/location for a medical facility, physician office, or independent equipment test places (i.e.: MRI, CT Scan, X-ray, etc.) probably has a venue of surprise – in barter system's value. Swapping location for services, equipment, and accessibility to the public without high costs of hospital stays. Insurance companies, government medical coverage, and private independent medical needs could also benefit by bartering to save $$$, however it is not clearly definable - how" (2015, Reddock, L's opinion; 10:42 AM 9/10/2015 [Yahoo | ©Rakuten Loyalty | Privacy Policy]

{**money**} This creation for funds as payment or gratitude, for products and services, has growth into *mental-anxiety*, for a majority of the human-race. Statistics can be accessed in daily, weekly, monthly, and an array of periodicals plus Internet business and population references to the **IRS;** a better website might be the US **Census Bureau**. Not along in paycheck-to-paycheck scenario, the human-race of: *whites, blacks, reds, yellows, and a vastly but unrelated-people, of identifiable-colors* work in: <u>facilities, offices, professional, and nonprofessional employees, and in the privacy of their dwellings performing various-jobs</u>. They desire to be paid, for the lengthy and dedicated hours, to guide children, spouses, neighbors, and a slue of individuals with needs that would normally go undone. Funding, money, and bartering have become an overall acceptable payment, for most beings. I do not question that salary or bartered gifts, room-and-board alone; nor do I question the clothing, jewelry, awards, and recognition for dutiful or sincere job projections, for patients. I do question the worth, anticipations which can be forecast via projected research and references, as well as personal observations and experiences.

- *"Do we each receive our worth?"*
- *"Is their going to be a place, during an illness of in-depth concern when we are returned our services?"*
- *"Will incidents such as inferred with the early chapters of this book, become the foreseen future, as it had been for decades of the 19th and 20th centuries?"*

I shuttered to think of the answers the answers to my own '**<u>questions and concerns</u>**' on a local and then a global-level. In as much as I have found *and* agree-with - *salaries & supplies grab large chunk out of private & government funding* - second only to physical structures being built, to treat patients. <u>*Overhead costs*</u>, of upkeep and maintenance for facilities (everywhere to live, work, vacation, and are cared-for during illness) continues to rise; higher costs can be projected from demographics supplied, from previous spending to include: *structural-building cost, insurances, taxes, local area fees, and installation of utilities*. Writing the facts is not difficult. Envisioning such an undertaking for the care, of the injured, on short to long-term cycle, may determine a sway toward … forget it! With many facilities already built, in fairly decent structural condition - utilities, food supplies, personnel, and a crew of maintenance employees basically cover forecasted-funds, to function. There are numerous departments within facilities that have been included in previous chapters, all requiring salaries as well for their services or products. But, the funds issued as grants, loans, payments for services rendered (immediately or at an unknown time in the future) by: *patients, insurance companies, and our government,* seem to be ignored.

Analytical machinery, equipment for observation, and pharmaceutical supplies has continued to reach unaffordable levels not because of lack-of input, by contributions. Apparently, many facilities pre-spend for frivolous anticipated needs. Billions of dollars might be calculated over a decade._ Facing such knowledge available on websites and articles in resource centers, is public knowledge which frequently remains – in clear-view – with nobody inquiring, reading, thinking of what the articles have projected. Funds are never going to meet the full-desired potential for a product or service, because the doers will consider their 'self-worth' valued at many more dollars than the purchasing consumer. Negotiations for products and services unrelated to life-sustaining or healthcare should not be a determinant, of cost to patients.

Research has disclosed '*Health*' as well as '*Healthcare*' has taken a 360 degree turn forward; the improvements documented, between the late 1880s and late 1990s – are exuberant. Specializing in financial and legal matters has become an area distinguishingly separate and apart, from healthcare occupations; as the leaders and administrators reached peak performances, for greed of our funding systems; coins, currency, bartering each has a place in the world. Each also has a time to become a rationale of expertise not a negative pay-off often the final commitment by those in debt!

And to overcome or reduce that eerie fact of negative pay-off prepaid package deals opened financial feasibility, to the public ***give now and slide later!*** The agencies, associations, organizations, and investment plans for insurance coverage in a time of need turns into a stressed out contributor to patients, in the form of mental-anxiety. So why was: "***Medicare, Medicaid, Pay Roll Insurance Deductions, and a variation of each for contributions ... created and maintained to a failing process?***" Let's explore results I discovered:

… way back when before our time community centers were formed; no cost to locals….

During the 20th century, it was different. How many dollars per hour can be charged fairly, for the cost of chemicals, equipment, and genuine healthcare created an open mind? With anesthetics and specialists to administer the numbing chemical, to a patient, was the start-of, "*what's it worth to you?*" "***Is the gurney, operating table, recovery bed, and bedding important your health? Does it require for each patient to receive privileges that have created – demands – by all patients for electronically powered head*** *and foot movement?" "Medical Personnel hopefully, not Doctor Frankenstein, skilled and experienced licensed diagnosticians, technicians, physicians, nurses, administrators, environmental personnel, accountants, and office employees all have salaries; must all non-medical-individuals lives be worth <u>financial disaster</u> because someone of those, dip into the funds?"* It appears that occurs more often than documented, along with five finger discounts by non-impoverished employees and totally disgusted patients; patients not upset with the ambiance but the lack of adequately shared-staff.

Student medical-surgical, nurses, and volunteers receive no income. They in-fact finance the institutes, universities, and medical facilities. How come there are not enough funds. Professors are licensed physicians with fairly decent practices, contributing to their personal living and office expenses; as long an malpractice and other types of insurances do not rip'em-off. Students purchase books at extremely high-costs, to use during one or two courses; those books often are discarded or sold at discounts, to poorer students. Does than make sense to borrow loans for educational pursuits to purchase uniforms, textbooks, laboratory kits, on-or-off campus residences, and hit yourself over the head with ripping yourself off down the road, upon graduation when those student loans must be repaid? It occurs at major educational facilities worldwide. Students are actually encouraged by professionals to do so, to deploy their future expenses. Hello, that is neither logical nor feasible in any way?!? *"How can paying $150.00 for a book that will be of reference in the future, swapped or sold at half or more that half its face value, become financially – a saving?"*

Understanding the rationalization for strategic-business preparations is an **<u>Accountant and Banking 101 class</u>**. Never, ever give-away anything of value, especially when you borrowed the funds to purchase whatever. There are no charitable financial-gains; and personal gains are not achieved by self-defeatist actions. Depriving one's-self of the value you borrowed to purchase reference, creates a self-denial which is not going to: *put gas in the car's tank, food in the refrigerator, contribute to your health or life* *insurance; so, orientation days' before classes begin might include 'how to become the man or woman of your dreams in medicine, without becoming a mental-financial lunatic,'* it may enhance tomorrow's youths desire to begin a self-worth flight without a financial fight which many educated individuals learned, will not be won at the end of their schooling.

Numerous students, in a variety of professions will have $20,000.00 to $50,000.00 of loans to pay; no matter how menial the interest rates, surmounting costs might decrease too slowly, for many to ever feel a financial peace-of-mind. And, worst that studying, financing through borrowed funds to maintain learning facility and its patients, does not ever end. There is no limitation to the research and personal interests, as I have come to find once returning to college, more than once.

Locally and in the Broward County Public Library System tack a cost for patron desires:

$.10 for a piece of paper to print from the computer's
printers
$.25 fed equipment to copy, whatever needs to be verified

Furthermore, business & propriety owners - along with tenants - contribute with rents. Small but valuable money is expected to open the door, for a *free-service. It doesn't occur! Indirectly, in an off-beat sort of the way, Internet access is free; however free computer-users assume it to be, forget its cost is attached, to monthly or annual fees paid to an Internet service provider (**ISP**) by: computer literates, businesses, students, and beginner level 'fun and excitement seekers'.*

It does not take a brilliant-mind to analyze double-payments, to public and medical facilities. I woke up a few decades back then in the 'thank goodness 20th century' and I became frugal; no longer because I was financially poor. Frugality arose for me when the first property owner's tax due estimate arrived. It arrived two or three months in advance of due-date with an itemization of what percentage of the payment goes 'where' and 'why.' That probably sparked my interests, into financial-concerns for no longer rising and overly reported medical costs to the elderly, poor, disabled, and wealthy. That property tax estimate opened my eyes, ears, and you name any senses unexpected to be imbedded in my mind and you gotta-know each came instinctually-prepared to critique' all correspondence from the government. That ricochet of instinct brought curiosity as to how come I have to pay for Fire Department, Emergency Medical Treatment or Teams? I am not burning anything nor will I permit myself to get sick.

Well, the list of how come and why didn't reduce the payments; nor do I complain too much but when push comes to shove, and rising costs exceed the average pocket – then I want to know why? And, here are the reasons; actually, only a few. You all can research an abundant reference in any place or book you like. You'll become as hostile or well informed with zillions of *unanswered* **questions**, as you learn more about the rising costs, interest rates, stock market shares purchased in and out of medical industries, and the cost of each frivolous purchase left in the back of the refrigerators of many houses … to be discarded into the waste bins. But for now the following list can be verified on the Internet, through periodicals, and human-resources throughout numerous local and global avenues.

Research and Reference Libraries: This was stated as student costs at thousands of dollars. A college student furthering their education can also incur thousands more, aspiring towards a Master's and Philosophy Degree also. So, their financing is the primary starting values, for all of the start-up of costs to patients. However, long-term upkeep and maintenance of structures, once the mortgages on the establishments erecting has been met, thousands of repayment dollars would appear applied else-where; it also appears at that point, a clear of liens by financiers creates additional funds, free and clear to be applied toward lesser things. But, it rarely is documented as a clear sailing, for the administrators, whom claim near-poverty for their dwindling facilities. Hmmm…!

Office Visits: This topic of concern varies from $50.00 to several hundreds of dollars, depending upon the location of the office; having nothing to do with income. Apparently a poor family would not be living in a wealthier area. However, with the

Medicaid funds from the government's contribution to statewide healthcare, a majority of the public turned into seasonal paupers during the 1970s to 1990s. Hey, have you ever heard the vulgar but true-to-life expression: "***If you can get the milk for nothing, why buy the cow?***" Americans are not stupid several are tightwads; more than several. The US Census Bureau's online (Internet) website reveals horrifying statistics of demographic data, according to: race, gender, region, and age. Another, hmmm…! In a compact view, there are not only 12 to 15 billionaires listed annually, in periodicals; here, in our vast country there are a minority group of paupers, at a ratio of between 1 to 100000: in the south and Midwestern states. This numeric ratio can be estimated according to the census reports submitted to include New England, Southwest, Northwest and all other areas with a ratio slightly lower; 12 to 100000 are near-pauper households. How can they not be accepted by Medicaid, United Healthcare , and local agencies, to keep the country's young and elderly - well? Somewhere between the young and aged remains that so called working public; those individuals are forced (politely), to contribute of payroll deductions, for their families. Something seems weird to me. Co-pay is often noted at receptionists' desks, of offices, stating you pay for the visits or you can leave; how come when $50.00 to $75.00 per paycheck has been allocated towards health insurance. Co-pay is $10.00 to $25.00 in many offices; but why pay for insurance that not does insure office visits, during an illness. When a person is healthy they receive an ***annual*** *free-physical*. It seems to me, there should be no cost unless a hypochondriac repeatedly has imagined ailments. There is a problem possibly overlooked, that hypochondriac patient might be psychologically impaired or threatened by someone. Such a patient (or person) requires specialist care not primary physician office visits; more times than average, potential-patient within insurance plans. I might think incorrectly. Then again, I have found through conversation others have similar thoughts.

Consultations: $75.00 to astronomical costs, depending upon type of physician, therapist, etc.

Examinations (including biopsy and laboratory tests): ***Don't ask!*** My spouse required a biopsy to detect a possible tumor within a bump on his nose; that cost Medicare over $1500.00. It was, benign! I cannot believe: a slice of his bump, three sutures, a swab of salve (twice), two band-aids, a sit-down on the reclining chair, for the procedures and evaluation, where the biopsy was performed created high costs. A prescription for antibiotics was issued, separate and apart from the cost billed to Medicare the first time. A second and third office visit was billed at an additional $250.00 each time; that cost did include: suture removal. Very strange!

Referrals: This piece of paper stating you need to be viewed by a physician, technician in a laboratory, and any combination of analytical evaluative random or pinpointed criteria, costs Medicare $0.00 except for the cost of the initial Office Visit; however, Medicaid, Insurance through Pay Roll Deduction provide a fee for authorization and bill the state and/or insurance companies. Private Funding $10.00 to $25.00. I am not continuing with the costs of receiving adequate signatures, for higher-intelligent means by those more familiar to what might be wrong with the average - patient.

Specialists: Can the idea of insatiable events with this category. There are more specialists than there are titles, for one or two groups of individuals in conference to bring to mind. However, we do need them, for brain surgery, reconstructive surgery, oral surgery, spinal and every systemic malfunction … to our bodies. Furthermore, as much as their expertise is required, I question not the statistically escalating from acceptable fees to beyond astronomical insane costs; fees paid (or billed from these offices) frequently are for consultations. Many consultations analyze and compare primary healthcare data, laboratory tests results, and evaluate the individual's future needs. It should be but not always is stated upfront, specialists do not always perform the surgical procedure, required to remove or repair a patient's condition. Costs…ha,ha,ha.ha! Yes, I am laughing to myself because a Plastic Surgeon's receptionist quoted the first visit at $250.00, plus seeing the doctor and being evaluated as a candidate for reconstructive surgery at anywhere from $550.00 to whatever; everything concentrated facts with realistic potential outcome, of the desired or required procedure. Well, that damn near could have reversed constipation to diarrhea had I have been a low-bowel patient. Fortunately, I stopped considering such frivolities. My scars can stay because not only would the current rate of specialist fees blow me away, the physical discomfort, pain, and long weeks awaiting the end-result might may me need a psychiatrist to cope. One time way-back when I found out, specialists arrange for surgeons to perform a good number of surgical procedures, patients assume are to be performed by their primary or very, extremely expensive specialist. Doesn't my input make you feel secure? It not only causes me insecure thoughts, this book had to be set aside since 1999 before I could allocate personal time, for revising and editing with removal of jargon and replacing it with actual facts, estimates statistical data or reference, for readers to seek their own knowledge.

Emergency and / or Admission: No, I can barely believe the costs for a minor injury, in an emergency room; its reasonable if you do not stand to lose a finger, extremity, physical mobility, and of course your desire to continue breathing. Hmmm…! {***hmmm…!*** has foreshadowed many aspects of writing for me}. It depicts a breathless moment in time, to encapsulate my deep-concern for my future, yours, and those silly but adorable domestic animals and plants, humans focus upon as silent-partnerships – to convey fears, without being gossiped about, from one ear to another, and so on, etc. But, really, the costs for a fracture (to be set or reset) at least $3500.00, that's if it is a simple procedure; let's not contemplate a smashed or multiple fracture of an extremity that has astronomical fees. Major emergencies frequently viewed by the team in hospital facilities, are delivered via ambulance, EMT, and possibly local police-fire rescuers. If you can't drive there, have a pal or spouse bring, then you most definitely will be treated above and beyond your imagined dreams. Yes, you'll be billed for every minute of every breathing minute, by all of the above – that were within a 2 feet radius of you before and after deliverance into facility. Tests, examinations, evaluations, diagnoses, prognoses, and please do not forget the ever necessary monitoring of such major importance – vital signs by a skilled but not truly accepted or considered to be professional. Laboratory and Radiology datum will become the beginning of a charting documentation, with half as many pages as this book prior-to being admitted directly for a few days care. Well, do I have to estimate the cost? Begin low - $1500.00 and go from there. The only cost that I have never seen on a billing statement was for a glass of water. Once I was billed $13000.00 for a two or three day stay in a hospital. They damn near gave me a coronary when that bill arrived a few weeks after I was home. Okay, they saved my life. Yep, at a cost of nearly killing me when a registered nurse, refused to observe the intravenous dislodged from the vein. The fluid in the plastic bag with some medication to get me back into good health was curing the bed-sheet and floor as it dripped from the covering needle band–aid. In the wee hours of one of those days, a nurse must have thought I was sleeping; she decided to inject, into that intravenous tube – a lethal substance. That same wonderful medical care facility issued via injection an antibiotic – of which – I had informed the numerous questioning professionals when asked, I had been told in my childhood I was allergic to. So, shame on me for not making payments, right…ha,ha,ha,ha! I do not think anymore needs to be stated within this section other than once before I had been treated for a similar upper respiratory ailment in full EMT delivery to an emergency room; the financial cost was 75% cheaper. I was treated as though I were god's gift to mankind or womankind. The staff monitored without injuring me more. So for me, a prelude to the rip-off in an ailment not faced in my childhood, I was the lucky one. *"Will I be as fortunate in the future? Can anyone be 100% certain their lives will not be harmed, by those charging them by the minute, hour, or day?"* Again, I'm pretty dumb when it comes to forecasting projections, from what I have experienced; some observations seem to have developed into dangerous pathologies, '*put on the blinders*' and don't look back. The limited included references have basically been covered within the first few entries. Although each of the following infers a patient can received great care, high costs will continue to rise upon the educated public and private sector; not because of need, lack of patients, nor the maintenance of facility structures and development of modern technological diagnostic equipment. Cost will rise because "_we_" the public and private sector will shy away from frivolous daily healthcare , after reading this book for a brief time. Such starves our facilities, and students will decline medical professional fields, for: **_accounting, legal, managerial, and custodial occupations_**.

If you are one of the few actually careless with your personal health, become debilitated by an unforeseen accident, give birth to a baby or multiple babies, and regretfully if you are a statistic between, golden years to graveyard, requiring long-term care, the following may encourage you to stay well.

(24 hour a day medical team care)

Surgery: includes too many procedures to mention, to mention a few: C-section, natural birth, heart-failure, respiratory inflammation, renal blockage, upper or lower intestinal disorders, amnesia, trauma as in shock from a blow to the head during a vehicular accident or the like, and replacements for hips, arms, legs, heart, kidney, or a slue of other types of transplantations of organs, start thinking $15000.00 and many more dollars as the list below develops patients into well-adjusted or acceptable individuals (by their peers).

Dietary (preparation, serving, and monitoring): from personal experience, well, how can I describe being issued a menu that you need not shop for, prepare meals, serve and cleanup after consuming pretty good portions? For many modern facilities, professional culinary dieticians and assistants create more meals than the average household could image, with more regular and special diet plans prescribed by physicians. Well, there are not many complaints or frightful experience within this area. The cost – most likely part of the daily admission fee – not itemized on any of the billing statements I have observed or reviewed. A majority of dietary personnel not only do all that sweaty-kitchen cooking, it contributes smiles as they serve pleasant or miserable, crabby patients. Every household could use a professional dietician with such dedication, I think - do you agree?

Rehabilitation/Occupational Therapies: are based upon an injury's treatment, required to adjust to the usage of prosthetic devices (external or implanted); frequently is elderly patients slipping. Fracturing a limb or skeletal-muscular supporting area on their body, they incur normally limited rehabilitation, for minor repairs. However, learning to function with artificial limbs takes time, practice, at astronomical costs, becomes disheartening. Furthermore, according to the US Census Bureau has reported injuries to contractors for construction includes: **electricians**, **masonry**, and **builders in a wide-array of architectural developments of dwellings to shopping malls to vehicle enclosures and the like** at 4,000,000+ injuries during a four year span of time, in the US of A. I may have very likely misread or misquoted the statistic or time span; however, the following is a direct copied and pasted reference page, of a research segment on April 5th, 2003.

Standard Industrial Classification - Claims Closed in 1999 - Some of the industries with large volumes of claims was: *Trucking and Courier Services Personnel Supply Services, Nursing and Personal Care Facilities, Eating and Drinking Places, and Hospitals."* *Industries with high average cost per claim include*:

- Nonresidential Building Construction (around $6.9K per claim)
- Motor Vehicles & Equipment (around $6.6K per claim)
- Paper Mills (around $6.7K per claim)
- Plumbing, Heating, and Air Conditioning (around $5.3K per claim)

All of whom injured *on-the-job* not only requires care, medications, and rehabilitation; occupational therapy is the alternate training, for injured and those born with birth-defeats. The *Occupational Therapy* field of medicine although not actually a medically professional field, is closely-knit to rehabilitation. Training those that not diagnosed as being acceptable to society's persnickety holier-than-thou attitude, require both physical and psychological therapy to adjust in both aspects of their future. It ain't easy! It ain't cheap! It ain't pretty! Yet, there are hundreds of thousands disfigured, not diagnosed, consciously aware they are perceived as being *different*. Many are unable to cope with such difference. Others, adjust; living in sheltered or communities provided through their previous or current contributions, by insurance and/or statewide growth and development centers. Supposedly, the anticipation that 'like-live-alike' will decrease staring; inquiries which offend disabled, handicapped, blind, and others '*different human-beings*.'

Another topic of not much noted: Worker's or Workmen's Compensation. Employers fund this program, for the employees, it is an insurance; employees terminated unreasonably, laid-off, and medically *on-leave* can often receive a percentage of their weekly 'earned' incomes – if they apply and are prepared to accept employment. "***How the hell can someone be prepared to work when hospitalized, in rehabilitation or occupational therapy, and at times undergoing psychological stress conveying random emotions and gut-feelings or paranoid?***"

Whatever, some lucky individuals collect *legally*. Others *rip-off* the program's funds. Numerous fraudulent claims are detected, others, cost employers *hundreds-of-thousands* of dollars. As for a percentage of eligible individuals there is small percent of applicants rejected. Those turn to public assistance, food stamps, and Medicaid to afford minimal daily-living expenses; many are also rejected. Others retrained without medical facility relationships, by professionals truly requiring a specifically educated addition, to a company. The cost for the training and employment costs the state and county tax-contributions by everyone employed. Somehow, many of the contributors cannot themselves receive, lest they are hassled by the applications being rejected and heard – in special group evaluations. It's a messy future. There's been nasty history, and for many individuals there is no end to their turmoil. And for the few that are able to cope with the frustrations of a free-society, increased premiums to barely live and die can proud to be not worth the aggravation. Perhaps that is why the crash during my grandparents era led otherwise sane individuals to commit suicide, as their investments and insurances were wiped-out by financial disaster caused by World War I, World War II, and those wars of my life-time during the 1950s, 1960s, etc.

Home Healthcare and extended: A blessing in disguise at times has turned into nightmares for those in need of minimal assistance. However, as a former geriatric care contributor through both facility and private duty employment, I was often welcomed. Furthermore, it is not the visiting aid, attendant, nurse or other professional receiving high-fees; mostly it is agencies, directing me there, you here, and the cycle of employment goes along as smoothly as possible. Restrictions bother me at times. I was unable to transport a patient with one agency, to a doctor's office, grocery store, pharmacy, bank, and on an occasional outing. There were insurance-related conflicts that would have concurred in the event of an accident or something. How ignorant. In the 1970s home care ranged from $75.00 down to $25.00, depending on the level of expertise or professional skill. *Hmmm...!* Too many elderly, disabled, and physically repaired but unable to obtain employment of litigations, documented how much pain and suffering a patient incurred [via monitoring with specific equipment]. Often physical distress was factually; yet, patients are as knowledgeable as many caregivers; they fake their injuries pain and psychological effects. Such contributes to the rising costs of care. It also diminished employment by reduced skilled workers, unable to detect the phony patient. It happens.

Pharmaceutical Costs (in and out of facilities): In my neighborhood there are pharmacies in nearly every grocery store, sundry shop, and practically on every once vacant corner lot. Walgreen's, Eckerd's, CVS, and others established online patient databases globally. For this particular book, I shall focus minimally on the where and strategic store-locations; because every business needs a consumer, client, customer, you name it and business cannot survive single-handedly. In medical facilities, numerous pharmaceutical departments were created to accommodate in-house patients. Once the patient is released for home or a facility for extended (long-term) or additional (temporary) care – written prescriptions flood the markets.

As news-reporters conveyed malpractice litigations with in-depth columns and ferocious need for reform to the public, greater demands on local healthcare once turned into traumatic experiences, brought less tension – in several regions. Solutions have not only appeared as a placating to irate patients; improvements became breathtaking, in a sedateful way, to professionals and their patient rosters. Volunteer employees and failing equipment re-established for necessity of both creations. Funds were not available for repairs or additional supplies, leading to many centers locking the doors. Those financially capable to remain open, through the turmoil of the 1970s and 1980s found inventions of medical equipment for both patient diagnostics and rehabilitation, superior; surpassing the lull revived a dying breed of scientific men and women.

Emergency Rooms of hospitals both local and within the realm of major, recognizable universities; patients once turned away or set on gurneys in loud, noisy, and brutal halls because of lack of funds took on a newness. EMT's were told to bring non-life-threatening patients to county hospitals where overcrowding occurred, each day and night of the week in the 1970s and 1980s; in the 1990s, a revival of care or local concern arose. Medicare and Medicaid merged, into a no-longer divided level of elite reduced to paupers' needs. That unification in the medical industry created schools to develop affordable student-insurance; more than one plan was available to prevent students from being discriminated against because their household's did not thrive financially. The obligation of healthy adolescents was the platform for aspiring politicians both locally and nationally; including presidential candidates. With strong family values projected, placing a gamble on early healthcare , to future generation's foreground did not suffer, it excelled.

Articles available in libraries and resource centers globally joined parents, not in unity of fellowship, merely in child-care and preventive illnesses with each child being able to have any care without hours in waiting rooms. Reducing stressful emergency scenarios parents no longer were forced (as in primitive times) to observe their young bleed, cry, and vomit as physicians were examining only the financially or well-dressed patients. These *excerpts* from **Medical Economics** and other **Infotrac Search Bank** reports, displays a fair amount of knowledge, just a small amount of the available data to inform the public, of the high cost of living well.

[1]*At long last one conversion factor only.*

Internists and other primary care physicians whose conversion factor has generally been smaller than the one for surgeons, have been lobbying, for the unified factor for a long time. Now they've got it. Next year the same conversion factor will be applied to all doctors.

Even though growth has been in the 2 to 3 percent range during recent years, it's unlikely to remain that low, even though it's unlikely to reach the double-digit percentages of the 1980s.

As for its impact on the average practice, the 37.13 conversion factor is being analyzed by the AMA's Center for Health Policy Research, among others. The Center's preliminary findings indicate that GPs and FPs will get a boost of more than 5 percent and internists will see increased from 6 to 9 percent, depending on subspecialty. But surgeons will take it on the chin. Cardiac surgeons, for example will suffer a payment drop of 7.7 percent.

If CBOs best guess proves true, however, doctors aren't going to be happy. Under the old law, by CBO estimates, the average of the three conversion factors would have declined to $35.66 in 2002. But under the Balanced Budget Act, the new single conversion factor will drop to about $32.63.

*"**Ninety percent of the political resources physicians spent during the past legislative session were directed at the practice-expense issue,**" say Doherty.*

Congress opted BBA to delay the resource-basing of practice expenses for 12 months [till Jan. 1999] and to require that it be fully implemented in 2002. In general the don payment will shift money from in hospital procedures to office based services. While the down payment won't save or cost Medicare anything – it's what folks in Washington call Budget Neutral; it will redirect about $390 *million, or about 1 percent of Medicare expenditures for physician services. Again, surgeons will lose; primary care doctors will win.*

*According to AMA, cardiac surgeons can anticipate a 10 percent drop in their payments, and radiation oncologists can expect a 9.6 raise. Others will see a change somewhere between those extremes. "**The range of payment changes is large but not unprecedented in the six year history of the RBRVS and the Medicare payment schedule.**" Says the AMA.*

[Already in affect and has many Medicare recipients quite confused and financially depleted from the 1980 to these 1998 years] Medicare in the years ahead keeps no secret, if legislators passed a law that forced seniors into HMOs and other managed-care plans, there would be hell to pay. Congress dares not tell the elderly what to do. Its only choice is to open the market and hope that new managed-care alternatives can cost seniors away from fee for service.

A change in the way HMOs payments are calculated is also likely to boost managed care. Under the previous law, HMOs capitation rate was tied solely to local fee for service spending. But the BBA established a minimum rate $367. a month per person in 1998 and a formula that considers national as well as local FFS expenditures. Next year, a region's capitation rate will be based 90 percent on local FFS fees and 10 percent on national averages; in 2003 the basis will shift to 50-50. All-in-all the budget act will increase HMO payments in rural America (where monthly rates now are often less than $300. per person) and in some poor urban areas. That in turn will encourage managed care to move into markets that it's ignored thus far.

In the past HMOs have lured seniors largely by offering preventive health services. But under the new law, FFS Medicare will cover mammography screening, Pap smears and pelvic examinations, annual prostate cancer screening, colorectal cancer screening, diabetes self-management, bone density measuring and some vaccinations. With what CBO estimates to be $4 billion of preventive healthcare offered within FFS over the next five years, some seniors may decide there's little reason to cast their lot with managed care.

The medical savings account, another AMA favorite is being given a trial run under BBA. No more than 490,000 individuals may sign up and the program is to be terminated at the end of 2002.

Two options would free the wealthy to spend more money on healthcare and allow doctors to take more money from beneficiaries. But will the options work? In what's called private fee for service Medicare, indemnity plans, which have to cover at least the same services as traditional FFS Medicare, are expected to offer additional services to attract customers. Beneficiaries can see any doctor and the plans not the federal government, determine the fees paid to doctors. Physicians are allowed to balance bills up to 15 percent over the plan's fee schedule, rather than 15 percent over the FFS Medicare. It's assumed that both the fees to doctors and the premiums for the private FFS Medicare plan will be substantially greater than those in regular FFS. Out of their own pockets, beneficiaries will have to pay the difference between Medicare's contribution and the cost of the premium.

Related Article: Crackdown. Congress tries to get tougher on health-law violators. The harshest provision in the act is the one that creates a civil monetary penalty, triple damages plus $50,000 per violations of the Medicare and Medicaid anti-kickback law. Some lawyers have suggested that this provision shows that Congress is in the mood for a hanging when it comes to fraudulent healthcare activities. The penalties are tougher than those for other civil disputes.

Related Article: Who's taking care of the kids? States get federal funds to improve children's health insurance programs. Poor Adolescents defined as those under 19 whose families are below 200 percent of the federal poverty level. "Over the next five years, the states are to get $24 billion, sufficient to give 5 million *adolescents the access they need for affordable health insurance," according to Sens. Edward M. Kennedy, D-Mass. and Orrive Hatch, R-Utah*

In general a state may use its money to extend its Medicaid program to more children, to purchase health insurance from the private sector, to contract directly with providers or to develop another scheme that meets the approval of HHS. The BBA require the standard for the money to be equivalent to that of Blue Cross/Blue Shield.

Another interesting article filled my interest about Medicaid on Hospital & Health Networks.

[2] *The gridlock-ness monster; the governors; proposal to save Medicaid from itself is going nowhere fast.*

The American Hospital Association and others oppose the National Governors' Association plan to permit states to reduce their Medicaid matching portion by 20% while continuing to receive the same amount of federal funding. {I wonder ... WHY?}

Commentators extolled the governors as heroes for breaking the Medicaid deadlock that had played such a large part in derailing last years' GOP balanced budget drive.

Under pressure from big states the NGA was proposing to let states cutback their Medicaid matching share by 20% without losing any federal dollars. {I wonder ... HOW?}

The AHA and other provider groups argued that the plan would eliminate provider protections, including the Boren Amendment rule – that payment must be "reasonable and adequate" and the right to sue states in federal courts if rates are too low. {I wonder WHICH provider groups?}

The offers from the NGA would cap federal payments to states based on previous costs and future growth, and hand states much greater flexibility in determining promised continued eligibility for certain groups including disabled, welfare *recipients, pregnant women and adolescents in working poor families, and very low income seniors in nursing homes. It also offered savings to the federal government of $59 billion to $85 billion over sever years, etc. The proposed blueprint would reduce the Medicaid contributions up to $214 billion over seven years (by the Center for Budget and Policy Priorities, a liberal advocacy group).*

Many states are seeking speedy federal approval of their plans to implement mandatory managed care for Medicaid recipients. Fourteen states have such plans, ten more filed applications. Numerous states are requesting to get control of Medicare dollars, as Minnesota had, to care for elderly and disabled patients eligible for both programs.

It's questionable whether these moves will actually save money, given the possibility of unintended consequences like service substitution. States clearly need federal reform to make the shift from defined benefits to defined contributions that would more certainly cut their costs. But Ray Scheppach insists, **"all evidence is to the contrary."**

Included by tax-dollars are costs related to patients (temporarily or permanently) confined, to government and private facilities. Medicare, Medicaid and Insurance payments are allocated for much more than individual or group treatment. Self-analysis is a therapeutic technique used, according to the data I extracted from the following article:

[3] *Journal of Nervous & Mental Disease* – This article caught my eye because I believe patients are not always as dangerous to themselves or others; many detained wrongfully, for the income from any number of sources, including government funding. In particular, this article mentions a therapy that:

- Analyzed the relations between the patients' psychiatric diagnoses, their self-image, and the staff's feelings toward the patients. Staff at 17 treatment units for severely disturbed psychiatric patients rated their feelings toward patients, on a feeling check list twice a year for 5 years.

Patients were diagnosed on a few levels, the results show: *the patient's self-image was more important in influencing the staff's feeling <u>than</u> the diagnosis [but] that diagnosis and self-image were virtually independent in this respect. APA/PsycINFO.*

Groups or other Medical Insurances purchased can be deducted from salaries and some are not fully understood by the insured. The problems arise only when the policy informs the insured that it doesn't cover the total cost of some things. Medicaid has become a back fall for those patients' bills also. It may be a relief to know there is a money *fairy* when we need one, for some people; it bothers me to think, individuals just might not be able to afford to get well. It might be better to allow an ailment to linger, never to receive a billing statement because it would be too expensive to even think about paying. Most likely that is only one of the many reasons individuals avoid bill collectors.

But I ask: ***"Will there always be a money fairy for the medically needed?"***

One annoyance I think the average mature adult will agree with in all sincerity is when in a hospital, for emergency treatment, patients are visited by social workers. They are employed by hospitals, to inform patients of legal-financial rights. I, for one, when being treated as a patient under emergency circumstances leading to admission, to the hospital do not want to be questioned or informed about anything except how to feel better. Therefore, I assume others feel the same way. When questioned by anyone (at times even a doctor or nurse) makes me feel intimidated. I have been through it and during my ordeal process on a gurney, I observed other patients [particularly elderly] being questioned once the spouse or family member went home. Many patients can't handle situations during a crisis.

Individuals in a doctor's office or hospital surrounding somehow forget important things (usually) because they are afraid of jeopardizing the diagnosis. They hide what could be symptoms, to avoid additional or possibly unwanted treatments. Some patients require sleep and reassurance somebody will be there when a discomfort arises (similar to the one causing them to be admitted). Some questions by the staff in many facilities in my opinion appears as being – *harassment.*

I figure: *"A patient isn't going to run off with the plastic eating utensils and find the nearest pawn shop, for a big financial haul, right? Maybe a nice fluffy towel* [not in any hospital I visited or stayed in] *would fit under a patients hospital gown or jacket; I doubt it will match the honeymoon suite bathrobe or a neighbor's prison jumpsuit. A patient's clothing usually can't go over or around tubes in the arms, legs or other body parts for intravenous feedings, blood transfusions or drainage such as a catheter; all of which are usually started when necessary or during admission to the medical center."* Of course I know my husband: *"would take the damn hospital bed if I asked him – just before he was given an estimated bill."* Other than those few exceptions *"what the hell is the big rush for social workers to pry into a person's life, or a nurse or clerk to get a signed form stating 'you are you and you live at ### street' in the same damn city?"* It reminds me of sales person or insurance adjusters, for the other guy.

Back to reality, *funding is an important part of business.* Hospitals, medical centers, facilities and other companies require money. As if you couldn't figure it out yourself. *"So how come after purchasing a house, paying taxes for more years than the average home owner would like to admit, on property 'you' can't be accepted when you think you might be almost dead? Why can't those taxes you pay to the county or state along with all the other taxes be enough to let a person recuperate from some ailment, accident or situation without pressure? And why are individuals taxed for some things they never use or have previously paid and no longer require?"*

The elderly unless I'm stupid or having hallucinations, paved the road, for: educational facilities with or without dormitories, classrooms, theaters, libraries, laboratories, campus frat houses and more. Books and tuition, for: professors, teacher's-aides, advisors, counselors, financial wizards and news-media are salaried, through students' tuitions. Fees parents or grandparents have provided, to build the campuses or prepaid for relatives, made life easy for a few. The majority of students still borrow to increase knowledge and skills. Maybe, just maybe, I'm starting to sound rude, I did not intend to do so, but I think the average household in America, is taxed too many ways, and for too many things including medical care. There are taxes for furniture, electric for lights and power to see, cook and refrigerate perishables, to run laundry machines (in many private dwellings), somehow that's not enough. We're taxed for telephone connections, calls local and long distance; telephones purchased or leased have a tax.

It's beginning to look as if the brilliant American population is the stupidest, in the world *yet* foreigners think we are wealthy. How the hell can Americans be wealthy when most of what we do is pay bills? Many, many bills! Every month it's the same old thing: mortgage or rent, electric, phone, cleansing items, personal grooming stuff, home-decoratives (for holidays or special occasions, etc.); groceries (oh GOD) so many damn groceries. If we didn't buy groceries we'd have to eat out and that would lead to another tax on the gas we buy, to fill the tank of our vehicle to go to a restaurant. Before we even leave home most adults would have to a baby sitter.

At a restaurant we'd be seated and told our server would be there shortly and along comes that smiling face. The foods [*often not as hot as supposed to be nor as cold*], sometimes, unclean eating utensils on the table [*should have stolen the plastic utensils from some hospital*], beverages the server brings before meals, are to get us to re-order. Bill placed on the table by the smiling server who just added ***tax.*** We tip a server not for the service but so the person can keep a vicious cycle alive. A better title for this book would be: ***My analogy of 'how life stinks.'***

A recent refresher experience with hospitals and treatments by a staff of professionals and others, might dissuade others from becoming ill. I couldn't breath. I stopped smoking, its called cold turkey, without the assistance of a physicians care. By the third or fourth day with no cigarettes, I was a wreck. Breathing was difficult. The desire for a cigarette was neither major nor miniscule. I enjoy smoking cigarettes, especially with a cup of coffee after a big meal.

I thought I was having a heart attack; the pain was severe. Nobody was home so I called 911 and though how stupid. The female voice answering the call was wonderful, she told me to try to relax. As I described the feelings I had, I breathed as labouredly as possible – to survive. It was a frightful moment and eventually the emergency ambulance, EMTs, and I were en route to the local medical emergency facility. Well, a previous chapter described that first upper respiratory ailment, and the second. That first was an experience to push me following my dream of comparing hospitals' services to patients, and other criteria. The second time I encountered an experience requiring my spouse drove me to a modern, more equipped facility which he thought was going to be able to cure me. That experience [is the one that] nearly killed me. Not only mentally bestowing immediate fright; but by a direct physical negligence of a nurse. The second incident was a nurse attempting to inject something into my IV not much more to rehash.

Hospitals have been given bad-mouthed patient nastiness till many and I myself cannot figure how to remove, not the inadequacies but the idiosyncrasies. My main petty-aggravation is why get the signature before the service is provided. How important but the timing just is inappropriately designated; when someone is practically dying – that's not a good thing to pester 'em with. If signatures made all that much asset-value I know where I'd begin; I would like a signature of the cashier in the supermarket when I pay with my ATM Card. How would that look? My spouse's barber, clerks in postal courier type of services, and oh how about the gas station cashier? The pun-fullness may seem inappropriate in a seriously written book but there are times, not I alone become frustrated by standing in lines to give a mini-biography and sign for something that is mine [or whoever is in front of in back of me].

Fraud a concern of many patients, as they review billing statements for: *treatments, prescriptions, procedures, and laboratory examinations for diagnostic purposes and care.* Not only the poor family income is double billed; middle-class and the wealthy find their errors are annoyances, not easily removed. Credit reports, focus history, and reliability toward increased or decreased financial status. Standing firmly against a medical billing error, refusing to pay in full creates needless confusion, also difficult to rectify or clear away from a bad credit status or rating.

What can be done? The most valuable solution: "***Stay healthy! Provide personal privately funded insurance, including a reliable nurse or assistant to make notations of the procedures, and the many tacked on expenses, to make you better.***" Relying on me, you, and a professional team of specialists can be as foolish as it would be to: *diagnose a major illness, plead a legal case as the attorney, and develop a technique for improving world peace alone;* it cannot be single-handedly achieved with needed success. Maybe I am wrong but that statistics are slim!

Audits of IRS forms, Inspectors affiliated with state agencies and associations see what they are led to view. The old-adage: *"what you don't know won't hurt you certainly has swayed many individuals,"* to a realizations that we are often not aware of that which is directly in front of us. In some facilities only a court order can get an Inspector in, for an inquiry. This creates problems for complaints of misuse or abuse, by a staff member only recognizable, by sighting it. Patients somehow don't ask for the name of the person attending their needs; if they do, they often do not write down the name or remember it. Inspectors in preventive negligence need to be incognito, for periodic inspections. Government and private insurances are not the only funding providing patients the right to good care; ethics portrayed most recently has become the norm. However, during the 20th century, up the ladder to success was a primary goal, for many professionals and university graduates, in diverse fields of study. Furthermore, success was developed to help but at what cost, to recipients?

Patients in beds unable to ambulate suffer from pains of decubitus ulceration to hips, buttocks, heels, elbows, and physical extremities, modern technology has not made a dent in reducing the majority of patients. Tilting and rotating beds ease the discomforts; how did those huge bed sores occur? Prevention requires patient treatment similar to that of an infant in many long-term facilities. Turning patients may be time consuming but it increases blood circulation, to an otherwise listless body. When I was an aid we changed many patients frequently (every twenty minutes). Longer than an hour or two is okay for patients with minimal ulcerations, if they can move about independently; patients need to have blood circulation to restore their skin, to a healthier condition. Many patients are (skin-irritations that are funded with the costs of daily long-term care) supposed to be not only turned, exercised, clean from soiled diapers or assisted to a bathroom or potty-chair can be found with body restraints. The restraints prevent them from falling or roaming freely; does that make anyone think why? How much does it cost to move off a chair, walk to a room when a light goes on, and assist a patient – that's the job of a nurse, aide, assistant or anybody with a stitch of decency!

The movie **Oh, GOD!** With George Burns delighted audiences. Other fine actors and actresses have been successful in presentations, of the real world. Patient care for the most part has improved. Good or proper care in the 1990s has increased still there is room for more improvements. Other observations and thoughts I have from previous views are as follows:

In hospitals during the 19th and 20th centuries patients were treated with less dignity because there were rare documents, presenting guidelines to professionals during a short term as well as long-term stay. Documentations of written, acceptable care and treatment desired, for an individual's final time has created a better tomorrow. Yes a Living Will shortened by illnesses' stress a patient, and loved ones. This make for decreased sorrow knowing the patient decided 'what to do'. Historically relatives or loved ones were responsible to pull the plug, of life support; as the latter part of our 20th century derived patient awareness and the choices, suffering has become lessened as well. Do Not Resuscitate (DNR), another document for patients to sign, providing direction, of their final days, as to what kind of emergency treatment should or should not be administered. A good thing however, when a professional in a medical facility does not review patients' charted data, this proves to be a waste of paper. If life can be less painful as one nears death, by all means I would think it necessary to prevent painful moments. Funds to facilities, for experimentation often create painful treatment, unsuspecting patients. It makes me leery about what the future will be for: my husband and I, and others in years to come. Controversy over misrepresentation creates financial problems for many communities; it also opened eyes to the cost expected for a decent and painless stay.

Human Rights Groups want individuals treated *humanely.* Government wants costs of treatment to be fair. Professional doctors, nurses, aides, etc. want more money to live better. At a rate hike of 11% annually a patient can expect to be charged approximately $104.00 per hour, according to the math for a bill of $15,000.00 for emergency treatment followed by a few days in a hospital. Frankly, there isn't enough value to pay so much and still be sick after treatments, tests, diagnosis, and rest. Actually, there was a nurse that ignored my request to look at the intravenous needle, during a stay in Coral Springs Medical Center, which had stopped functioning because it was dislodged. Hmmm! Without liquids/fluids and IV medications there most likely is a prolonged illness.

The **dietary staff** probably had the only smiling faces, during a few hospital stays by me. Although eating food was not my problem, it [the splendor of the attitudes of food server] made me believe there were individuals that liked doing a good job. Bed Rest is the one thing that cures most ailments; often it is what parents and retirees need. In a hospital that's rarely going to be obtained.

Sleep might be worth $15,000.00 (or more in an electronic bed). {But} not when a simple aspirin is $1.50 or more. Let's face it, there are 100 to a bottle normally, at a cost of $3.00 or $4.00; the price of an aspirin makes for rip off head-on. This seems unfair to patients and their insurance; it seems unfair and quite ignorant of our government, to pay through Medicare and/or Medicaid insurances. Lots of things go on in a hospital facility; patients normally are unaware.

Service is one thing I believe that should be given with high standards and graciously, instead, out of sight/out of mind. Behind the scenes type of stuff include: lack of some employees doing less to maintain professionalism, avoiding responding to patient calling, and assisting patients with morning/night cleaning (of dentures, final bathroom needs, etc.).

Although paperwork, essential to statistical reference, for developments of improved patient care, treatment, and equipment require documentations, so is it necessary for patients to have nurses in reach. In the past 5 or more decades desk sitting prevented sufficient care while writing notations, which is a waste of billions of dollars, if patients are not being cared for properly!

Laboratories doing research on: Humans, Animals, and Plants are funded by government dollars, as subsidies for major health-related ventures. Banks provide loans if failure to repay might turn property and documentations over, often used as collateral. Banks and private lenders finance corporations that appear/seem capable of repaying at high interest rates. Compliance with funds received would be adequately dispersed, for success as well as experimentation, to created and develop a product or regimen to improve disease.

Facts, research and fear verify for lenders (i.e.: government, banking and insurance companies) that assisting research projects can increase taxable incomes, from a successful product as well as systematic treatment change from okay to much improved. Research statistics describes how-to administer a new drug, what can be expected and the probable negatively unacceptable side effects that may occur – in some patients. Experiments of plant-like byproducts are used as the foreground, of creating and developing a medication; it becomes available on a 'trial-basis' on laboratory animals primarily. Proceeding along to *human beings;*. frequently tested for diseases or miracle cures not currently reported or available otherwise.

Individuals in negative economic growth had during the 19th and 20th centuries sold themselves to the scientific field, anticipating a roof over-their-head, which may prove to be helpful. Individuals not admitted to a medical facility or laboratory receive compensation; a cigarettes or free drugs. During experimentation times those individuals life turns into hell. Their *hell* becomes a struggle to survive, and their hell becomes stressful on taxpayers' and the economy! It appears the more researchers progress intellectually, technologically, and advancements surface, to improve the quality of life, a burden not really wanted also arises.

Reading the book may be eye opening, however it does not include direct facts, required to guide individuals and professionals in a direction to decrease spending, in a particular area. Our internet provides statistics, facts, and avails currently inclusions. Demographically costs of medical help varies; ailments, patient care, and treatment should not vary. Low-income areas publish drained economies. Public universities and government-funded facilities during emergencies are incapable of handling the massive turnout of patients requiring treatment. A wide immeasurable gap confirms wellness is the farthest concern, in many households until a crisis. The increased aging population has grown rapidly, nearly tripling that during the turn of the 20th century; reproduction of offspring increases statistically almost of rapidly. Prescriptions increasing annually, to maintain a healthy body, specifically to the aging population in the United States alone will continue to rise, for all economic levels. Middle and low-income families cannot afford medications lest their household does without necessities, such as: food, clean clothing, heat and air conditioning, etc. Nothing stops at necessary needs, as each family has varying necessities *because* cutting out physical comfort does not help that true cause. What can be done is a query quite difficult to answer. It may be unanswerable....

Below: a notation copied and pasted website inferential, for readers to access their answers, regarding conditions often overlooked, by strangers. Another great and far more qualitative website to visit, for access to demographically escalating and most needy areas is: www.uscensus bureau.com

Demographics Data   US Census Bureau Records free information.

Schedule for Income, Poverty & Health Insurance Stats and ACS Results September 08, 2015

MEDIA ADVISORY The U.S. Census Bureau announced the schedule for the 2014 income, poverty and health insurance coverage statistics and the 2014 ACS releases.

The websites available all the time to the public can provide abundantly statistic and research documentations, each focusing upon individuals, families, locations, incomes, and so much more. Do not hesitate to ponder your locale first, then the surrounding areas, for a vast completion to necessary data most recently updated.

<u>5:15pm, Saturday, April 05, 2003</u> I visited the website of the US Census Statistics, the website provides data on webpages eliminated a need for me, researching data, to verify personal skills. In this book's original reference I did not think to seek reported *statistics, facts, or demographics*. References were simplified; easily accessed just to get my thoughts in adequate but as a rough draft. 2015 years have come and gone with additional updates, revisions, and both negative & positive changes to the medical field, regarding patient care and treatment.

Faced with a desire to complete the project of 1999's primary book length data with comparison facts and correctly documented material because essential. Databases available to the public, developed into a knowledgeable guideline, after the primary roughly drafter book was set aside, as too complicated for me to complete. Printing it 'as is' did not conclusively provide ample nor valuable data; therefore that book was only book-bound and sent to many relatives, as a lifetime of my experiences and opinions. Not everyone wishes to read or create a book, so I did, on the topic of patient care.

Research on the US Census Bureau website brought a variety of data, pertaining to available <u>facts, figures, regions, and many demographics;</u> reducing my finds with where-to access additional data was the easiest aspect, for others to display their interests – more important to themselves than mine. ***Excerpts*** pertaining inserted have been noted, as referential inclusions. Understanding negligence's onset is affecting regional economies, racial discomforts, and over viewed lack of care, to patients. There may be considerable answers to unknown reasons such as: "***why***" a handful of employees display minimal regard for employer's and patients needs. Researching high-cost of medical care in itself creates high costs; however, illness per capita in the United States and globally can be identified, with potential financial decreased stress, by seeking the internet's communication available. Problems have narrowed to a halt, in facilities treatment as legal professionals develop strategic policies, collecting simple data/facts, and combining analyzed observations to government's problems reported. Legal aspects for prying:

financial departments, in-house patients, outpatients, and emergency treatments are available, in databases.

Investigators attempt to halt negligence for improved treatment. Their presence in facilities (i.e.: private, public, and otherwise prominent), under both governing prowess and independently to gather data, stand firmly, in a pursue to omit negligence. Employees, on call physicians, and administrative levels must be held accountable. Legally prowling with a realization of ***probable cause*** is projected during investigations; many gone without full knowledge of staff members, properly receive and report accurately activities within facilities. There are not as many contributing investigators and individuals filling databases; there are a handful releasing updates.

According to the census bureau's, an easy to comprehend process has taken place over a period of four decades during the 20th century. Specific facts are direct copies, pasted into this chapter, so I do not screw up my interpretation of the facts and statistics.

[4]*The Neighborhood Change Database is based on the geographic unit of the Census Tract. The Census Tract is the Census Bureau's statistical equivalent of a large neighborhood (with an average of about 4,000 people). You can select any of the four geographical levels:*

These population weights were then applied to the various 1970, 1980, and 1990 tract level NCDB variables to convert them to 2000 tract boundaries. The population weights were used to convert all variables based on counts of persons, households, and housing units, all counts based on subpopulations (such as black persons or elderly households), and all aggregate data (such as aggregate household income). Proportions (such as the proportion of Hispanic persons) were remapped by first converting the respective numerator and denominator values (Hispanic persons and total persons, respectively) and then recalculating the proportion.

Understanding how neighborhoods change is fundamental in addressing problems, and opportunities in America's communities; many individuals are not aware that data obtained from the U.S. Bureau of the Census cannot be used directly for these purposes,

...because: of many changes, in census tract boundaries and variable definitions between census years.

[5]*In the early 1990s, with funding from the Rockefeller Foundation, the Urban Institute made adjustments as necessary to create the first national data file with consistently defined tract level census data for 1970, 1980 and 1990. That file has since been used as the basis for important* research on how the nation's communities changed over three decades. *Rockefeller has again provided funding to allow the Urban Institute, to add 2000 census data to the file. GeoLytics applied their proprietary weighting tables, for 1970, 1980, and 1990 to carefully convert past census data, to new 2000 tract boundaries.*

The collaboration has drawn on strengths of both organizations and private citizens' contributions. It resulted in a product that is a significant tool for policymakers, researchers, and community practitioners interested, in neighborhood changes. Other affiliated documentations of statistics per capita and/or within regional localities can be accessed in the US Census Bureau, for instance: H-Demog: Business Information Alert, Coordinated GIS, Seattle Times.

"What makes the GeoLytics CD a quantum leap over census data on the internet is that it allows you to pull up demographic data of a series of geographic areas, a group of towns or neighborhoods, for comparable reference. The raw data to do those kinds of investigations was available before but building a database or spreadsheet to work with it was an arduous job. The GeoLytics CD makes it simple to export information to a database or spreadsheet, and you don't have to deal with overloaded servers and long download waits on telephone modems. I particularly liked the Neighborhood Snapshot feature. By simply typing in your ZIP code and street address, you can call up an instant and very useful, demographic profile of your neighborhood. You can also customize the

portrait to include demographic information, for an area within a designated number of miles." The Hartford Courant, Enter (Technology) Section, August 18, 1997

Medical Ethics has been the background for many to shield themselves. It had become a guise. Currently (1999, 2003, and 2015) ethics seems to openly project improvements, do to escalated costs within medical facilities. Often ethics refers to various aspects of words frequently used in written text and conversations; occasionally, ethics is not directly believed necessary in treatments or care received. Why?

Attorneys and the USA judicial system hear cases involving psychological and physical negligence as a legal halt; frequently, settlements are issued, to compensate patients. Does this procedure improve or negate the malfunctioning staff or facility's future wrongdoings? My beliefs continue with limited inference, of professional recorded documentations, filled with statistically unimaginable high-percents.

Geriatric dementia is discussed amongst greedy and wretched individuals whereby the aged requires or is coerced into custodial decisions, legally. Although it occurred in prehistoric centuries, the process has continually advanced, as incomes and wealth increased in families and businesses of vast success. In the 19th century horrendous, often unnecessarily painful surgeries were performed, for experimentations. I'd like to believe in the 20th century changes were legally prevented. How can prevention to the unknown take part, in a medical facility? That is the true judicial systems' global obligation, to the taxpayers, to professionals, and to patients. As horrors encountered during my childhood was not rectified, settled, or reduced - other adolescents have been subjects similarly; abused and neglected patients not only the senior citizens (who have stashed a few miserable dollars), to live in comfort. So in this 21st century, again investigations privately as well as federal funded observations must continue, to prevent and to repair neglectfulness.

Many adolescents and senior citizens are in similar categories because of legal age recognized as acceptance or questionable to undertake self-sufficient care; therefore, many are ripped-off financially. *"What else can be done?" Seek out legal advice during a*

131

threat, is not always time-faithful. Do not settle with a diagnosis that has not completely in your medical history. Ask friends, neighbors, family members, or clergy, when stress surfaces; instinct is normally the body's way of questioning something not right."

Euthanasia - assisted death; good and bad points. In the United States controversy legally is communicated and documented, of irrational decisions. The topic is not one I believe in, personally; furthermore, it seems to be one of the decisions for others to become involved with better understanding. Controversy religiously, legally, and morally debates have been reported. Over the internet individuals can access websites, known for assisting in death. Here in the USA there are several states that have approved assisted-death. By a totally lost individual with nothing to live for <u>except</u> pain, stress, and an incurably prolonged disease the judicial system hears requests, by attorneys, for patients; the judge has the right to approve or deny the cry for euthanasia.

From my standpoint the concern becomes a problem that does not merely touch one person. Euthanasia effects young, old, black, white, and every human being en route to their religiously or worshipped leader, i.e.: God, Allah, Satan, or whomever's ***country in the sky*** – might to be evaluated for their specific state-of-mind, before permitting such an ending. A valuable point for patient, insurance company, government, loved ones and others might be: "*removing one human being facing a future of pain or misery (of a comatose life) without realistic promise of a decrease or cure, in a reasonably anticipated time limit*" creates a subtle but major relief, if only in my opinion. The negative point or aspect of putting a patient to sleep (as one might do to a family cat, bird, dog, etc.) is: *<u>public enemy number one get smeared throughout the city</u>*, where this horrendous but peaceful-end to a miserable future, occurs. Nasty ***labels*** are placed upon the family members either by society or self-inflicted. Labeling comes from the '***guilt-factor***' most individuals have been taught, from day one of their communicable life throughout their educationally, structured studies or civil lifestyles.

In an oddball way I'd like to live out my life till I no longer can function mentally, physically, and make contributions, accepted or rejected, to others. Maybe 85 or so would be a good age to die; maybe not. Maybe, through technological & medical advancements, the improvements can prove worthy for individuals to live, to be older with more to contribute than: *opinions, books, and material things*, as gifts to loved-ones

In the articles I researched I have come to realize **Health Maintenance Organizations** (HMOs) connect economic interests to physicians, to the financial goal of the HMOs. I use this as an example because it has been over the last twenty years plus additional decades that HMOs became a number one means, for patient *self-preservation*, through physicians, nurses, and responsible administrative personnel. No matter how precautions are implemented, individuals will become ill. It is not till then, when all sorts of questions surface. Insurance companies of today (20thC to 2015), and the future may not be as lazed in paying for legal overtakes, by relatives, placing loved-ones asleep (euthanized) to omit stress, and related problems.

Although not included in medical ethics article, during the 20th century, there has been numerous **organ transplants,** permitting life to be successfully rejuvenated, by a patient otherwise incapable of functionality. The costs of ten to twenty per cent uncovered by insurance, affordable to the wealthy, for many years has hindered general household's medical coverage. It has been at the expense of patients involuntarily used, for the sake of experimentation, which has a 50-50 chance for success after surgical procedure.

Donors with desires for *their* body parts to be used for the improvement or life-sustaining situation, to mankind have made living tolerable for many. There are situations that have led ***impoverished*** parents to sell their children, for scientific exploration, to improve life for others also. Much of medical science's goal to heal has been abused, by villains, as they purchase human-guinea pigs.

Cadavers stolen by lunatic practicing physicians or others were mutilated for sick and selfish gratification *displayed in movies* such as: *The Portrait of Dorian Grey, Dr. Jeckyl and Mr. Hyde, Frankenstein, and the Boston Strangler.* Proving incidents of this takes guts, proof to prosecute, and to stop such viciousness. A chore movie authors write about and make seem easy, is projected through direction, utilizing both moral and legal standings; no producer wishes to be named in a lawsuit, for presenting slander. Public opinion cannot be shown in explicit negligence legally; it is considered an infringement of privacy. Criminal acts are often not satisfied, by proof to back up atrocities, in court that provide public opportunities to pursue beliefs in civil courts. Torts (civil actions), prove to be more reliable than criminal actions. Torts restore not only monetary losses rather it reiterates emphasis on the public believing our legal system works.

Genetic engineering has made gene therapy possible, availing cells to be observed and analyzed in laboratories.

Somatic cell therapy used on humans in the United States since 1990 (which affect only the patient) has been inclusive in cell studies as well.

Germ line therapy which has not yet been used in humans, would introduce genetic modifications not only to the patient but also to the patients' offspring, raising questions of moral acceptability, of modifying a genetic line. I wonder: '*Who authorizes such tampering? At what cost to society, financially, and morally?*'

An interesting point was written in the article aforementioned. It seems to have less respect or impact on society than the *American Medical Association Code of Ethics and the Hippocratic Oath* intended. Both *Code and Oath* stress the importance of confidentiality, the need to treat patients with dignity and respect; highly transmissible diseases such as: HIV/AIDS that pose ethical dilemmas. Some physicians have and will continue to refuse treatment, to patients with communicable diseases (i.e.: AIDS), to eliminate potential spreading the disease to others.

The following ***Torts*** pertain to civil wrongs, which in some way bring injury to persons or property for which the law provides a remedy, in the form of an award of a sum of money.

Malicious Prosecution the remedy for instituting – *with the intent to injure or harm* – criminal proceedings against the plaint

Negligent injury may not have been intentional; it nonetheless may be blameworthy because the defendant did not use reasonable care under the circumstances. Unavoidable injuries do occur and even thought a plaintiff is injured, if the defendant is in no way at fault, he or she is not liable. Accidents may arise from a variety of causes: *the failure of physicians or other professionals to meet the standards of their calling* (**Malpractice**) *and the negligent manufacture and distribution of defective consumer goods* (**product liability**). Most cases do not allow damages for merely mental distress. Large awards based on considerations led Congress in 1996 to enact legislation to "cap" product liability awards. The bill vetoed by President Bill Clinton in May, whereupon the U.S. Supreme Court continued to focus, effortlessly. Even though a case in negligence may be established as outlined above, the defendant may still defend on the basis of contributory negligence means that the plaintiff's own negligence or is some states, comparative negligence.

Contributory negligence means: the plaintiff's own negligence was partly the cause of the injury. If this can be shown, the defendant will win even though he or she was much more at fault than the plaintiff.

Conversion and more are included in the research. All of which are only surface damage physicians, attorneys, clients, and general public face and fear.

As for a phony *Tort*, money proves to be the enticement. When a judge sets a judgment it was appealed; often the appeal favored the poor mistreated. Patients complaining of malpractice or abuse were seen removing a brace, lost their mentally inactivity (displayed in a courtroom to gain sympathy from a judge and/or jury). Such cases led to higher costs, for physicians to operate a business in many communities. With failed discipline by a legal system such as United States', let us ponder these questions:

1. *What the hell the world will be like when old age is all individuals fear?*

2. *Will there be too high a cost for an emergency room visit when ill?*

3. *Can physicians become scarce, perhaps non existing during the aging years?*

4. *Are adolescents and loved ones in an emergency lack proper medical care?*

5. *How many individuals will trust any professional after bad publicity, during the 1970s and 1980s?*

And more to the point let us continue to grasp additional summarized activities to select for ourselves, which is best to plan to avoid problematic negligence.

Legal Actions vary from business-to-business, and complaint-to-complaint often leaving individuals to assume all will be aright when we reach a doctor's office, or an emergency room. The lawyer will know what to do, a judge will cast proper fines. Realistically, thoughts of anticipated relief is a façade, quite often. There is no guaranteed peace-of-mind. There is only *hope* that you get a professional with *ethics, knowledge, experience,* and *the skill* during your crisis. For those with commonsense the ability to realize professionals in or out of the medical field are *scientists* as well as *caregivers*; we must relate to their service provided. Professionals (of long ago), were looked upon with a high-level of respect when not being thought-of as ***quacks***.

The wealthy often paid enormous fees to have a physician eliminate an annoyance, or illness to a household or community. It was frowned upon as being *unethical* [but] it had benefits; an intruder or culprit with a difference of opinion or desired lifestyle may have converted a team of soldiers or others, to revolt against a wealthy leader. The world was safer and less frightening for evil doers, knowing their threat was removed. The wealthy remained in charge of townships, households, and family with staff members. In the centuries and decades long gone unsuspecting nice individuals were cautioned to beware, by the more informed. Verbal expressions only, could define the difference between right and wrong. Medical aspects depended upon the price a person could afford, to live as he or she chose. As of the middle of the 20th century came about after the wars things began to changed, drastically improved.

Modernization took over. Aircraft was accessible to transport military personnel and supplies to areas often unreachable, by vehicles. Hiking woodlands and swamps brought new diseases, for medics and trainees. Cures, used by native country folk, incorporated into the modernized medical studies, has not yet ceased to grow intellectually worldwide.

It has added to the variable treacherous danger and harm to others; at times, undetectably. The law protects both defendant and victim it seems; perhaps, in too vast an aspect with the primary guidelines of our Constitutional Rights. ***Where does that leave victims, which have no proof early-on and those damaged intentionally?***

Journalized thoughts and findings document regional *population patterns of human and other species* [animal and plants included], *diverse methods for diagnosing and curing ailments required quick disclosures* limiting disclosures to the public. In order for data to be introduced as ***verifiable evidence***, students in universities connecting abilities are made accessible through telephone lines, as well as cable connections to the internet, for legal systems, and medical research and development facilities. It appears a vast number of countries have telecommunications, permitting anyone with a computer in the office or home to contact the worldwide web; querying data requires no great skill, other than technological knowledge to access databases and search engines, regarding interesting and documented facts revised as well as historically compared to a specific time span. Inquiries often deter searches because there are hundreds of thousands of returns, for a query. To legally convey typed questions with as much detail available, creates success in s skilled transmission.

It amazed me when I reached a library in Canada, California Universities, and other states; and internationally connecting to a research center of a country, way out of my desired query. I thought this must be illegal, and I'll be accused of prying. After securing educational escalation, in my adult life I had come to realize there is no limit to access legally available to the public. It's all in the know how-to inquiry. Because I research both in resource centers, colleges, community centers, and public libraries there are no limits to the available information. How much of what I know, from where it was received, and the way it is represented in a document is an important legal aspect, of doing! Yes doing something correctly, for the betterment of mankind. Therefore, it is as important to train myself or anybody, in a competitive way as much as it is to pursue, independently.

Flex-sessions (Online-Studies) gives home ridden students an opportunity to advance educationally, occupationally, and to assess their mind's capacity to function in a technological venue. No matter how severely prognosis dictates otherwise, impossible individuals that truly desire advancement can even if they require assistance, from caregivers. Transmitting emotions, can assist in the reversal of a diagnosis that pertain to grimness. Verifying a patient's ability to relay information of conditions, either medically or personally being run-a-muck of opens the door for changes in areas of healing often swept under the carpet. Legally an important development for the judicial system, to fight silent harms; in addition, the enhancements of videos capturing activities can verify the individual, and the villain.

A personal computer can be an expensive investment; it can also become the life saving device, for many shut ins. Legally, faxing a document can be done only by consent of the person the information belongs to (or that has it in their possession). Computer communications can be transmitted without stealing the documents, by scanning originals into a computer, and transferring the image as attachments in an email. This may not be news to all the readers, it has proved to me that a million miles may stretch across or around the world but documentations can be verified up front, on a screen through a scanning device or camera attachment. Now if that ain't modern technology, in the 20th century then I don't know what other legal purpose a computer might be.

This 21st century has years to go to reach the future, for many senior citizens; it has to go beyond expectations, for those in educational primary pursuits, and even perhaps till the end – for newborns, as this 21st century has already attained 15 years. With each decade ahead, I may only live through two, three, or four. My theory that malpractice reported and cited in courts from the 1960s to the 1990s reveals individual physician guidelines, which were required, to prevent such allegations should never have been done to begin with.

Attorneys with dollar signs in the their eyes continue, to seek patients of automobile accidents; in emergency rooms squatters sit awaiting critical patients to be brought-in. Contacting greedy bosses for contingency agreements upon either recovery or diagnosed as terminally ill, by specialists, attorneys tend to benefit psychologically long before courts award $$$. There are many cases successfully won. Others lost for lack of proof or verifiable evidence, proving criminal intent. Efforts should be commended for over turning antiquated legal precedence into the public's view not condemned.

As for legal actions in regard to medical ethics, there will never be high enough standards, to practice or study on a recurring basis. It takes more than a few researched articles and documentations, to improve the physician-attorney-patient-connection. It takes decency on behalf of a world, not yet ready to come clean of: ***get rich quick desires***!

With knowledge of what had or can occur came the desire to stay well, for me and the over-all public. The ability to use skills to reference fitness and diets prevailed, displaying individual self-confidence. Studying personal or professional pharmacology and other topics, such as: *medicine and law*, led a general-educated public into the knowledgeable steps required, for self-preservation. Let's take a glimpse down a memory lane often avoided, for its connotations of shame, fear, suffering or ignorance [to reality].

1960s *Hippies* [also referred to as Beatniks] introduced *free spirited independence and flower children.* They wanted no physical warfare, murdering innocent individuals in or around the world many marched to Washington, for *American Rights.* Headlines and articles in some periodicals used slanderous and factual stories, to reduce the impact of the Hippie Movement to a mere outspoken view, of unfortunate teenagers. Musicians, actors, gurus joining together; revamping previous attempts to negate issues of their visualizations of truths and goals, for young Americans (and global recognition and equally), they developed phases of life suitable, for growth. Such occurrences and events led to confrontations and by the age-change from youthful flower power, to mature entertainers. Many relabeled by peers and admirers; no longer were *Hippies beatniks.*

1970s *Yuppies* (a branch-like sector of Hippies once degraded for their emotional desire to be free of *cold-blooded actions*) excelled. *Baby Boomers* it took me years to understand "*I*" was part-of that generation. *Social Security* and *Medicare* (prepaid by the working force in the 1930s, 1940s, and the 1950s) were big issues. *Malpractice* was introduced and overly drawn into - the homes - of millions, by televised newscasters and hungry attorneys - were like vultures; preying on the injured, to make public records of settlements (for a third of the court's decision), if a case was filed and won.

1980s *Human Rights groups* debated publicly and privately about malpractice cases pending decisions, in the United States. Patients lingering in a comatose status were being kept alive with technology, such as: <u>intravenous or gavage feeding as well as with tubes to cleanse both urinary and bowel tracts</u>; patients lived with minimal mental capacity according to monitoring of brain activity. Rarely expected to come around to being themselves' - their unconscious existence destroyed faith (for many) in scientific studies. Large sums of money paid to attorneys, to request judicial consent to discontinue all life-saving technology was usually wasteful. Emotions caught hold of community leaders, striving to make political stands. Some demanded justice and less stress for families from the conditions of the loved-one suffering. Scientific meandering continued beneath a guise: "*<u>there's always hope for a cure as guinea pig actions were performed in the name of human research and experimentations, to benefit mankind.</u>*" The world was stunned into facing reality, there is no-way **death** can be a solvent for tragedy.

Sexual assaults were brought to view mostly on children. Outrage led neighborhood to secure their communities. Police offered guidelines to working parents claims followed by reporters, not judicial center harassed and injured families emotionally. Less was done to put an end to bitterness felt in many homes. On a less strenuous note family togetherness thrived, for some.

Amusement Parks and Recreational campsite became affordable, for vacationers with children. Actors and actresses created and broadcast Fitness Videos as Health Spas, Fitness Centers, Community Screening Facilities and the like informed men and women of a bleak future, if they continued to eat, sleep, shit, and fart for the good life. By the end of the decade, everybody seemed to be returning for continued or higher education classes, once believed designated for formerly teen dropouts from high schools. Religious leaders, not overly popular gained family contacts projecting Godly thoughts led to clean living; it epitomized the worldly view for many families. Families joined the search of a better way to live and raise children. Adults stuck in low paying jobs switched roles. Adolescents gained an admiration and a macho image of men slid into the shadows by dual partnership, at home.

1990s Physician Assisted Death gave living a new outlook. *Individuals moving* away from cities because unhealthy air and conditions of housing, country dwellers tired of farming and horrendous bad weather, and distance between neighbors, swapped places. *The New York Yankees* won the World Series [1998] in a four straight-game performance. Living advanced to less friction, more understanding and considerations, by parents for the children. Working conditions improved along with the minimum hourly wage, to a fair level.

Life in general took a revolutionary step forward. The year 2000 was first brought into homes by silliness in cartoons. It was projected in the news and movies as being the most well unspoken topic, of current events. Indeed the year 2000 brings not only a new decade; it brings an entire century to an end as a neo-calendar view opens the minds of every living thing including, human-beings. With two years remaining the 20th century there is plenty to do in preparations, as the 21st century hits home filled with excitement for young and old.

In *Medical and Surgical fields of Science* there has been and probably will continue to be controversy; pains and aches, colds and trauma, births and deaths explored and documenting will follow the pattern of living, hopefully without the in depth experimentation of the centuries that have ended. The world may be a better place as a result of: *'outer-space'* and *'deep-sea' adventures.* Many explorations have led to knowledgeable ways individuals can benefit. Not from *gad-zillions of dollars spent on experimentation and exploration* of foreign areas but by using the strategy of brilliant and (possibly) obsessed individuals – provided such occurrences a path from daydreams to reality.

I can't determine anything other than what has been lived, and noted (by others or myself). I can however claim knowledge leads to actions. And realizing *knowledge includes statistics, facts, ideas, movies, news, sports data and more* information to improve or delete daily living. Often **knowledge** is stored in a variety of materials (i.e.: books, cassette tapes, periodicals, newspapers, microfiche, and computer disks), permits access to individuals seeks information. Information, of which, is not always clearly understood. It provides **dreamed aspirations** of a small percent of the world's population.

Some **knowledge** is not written, drawn, videoed or stored. **Life Experiences** is unknown because individuals in private sectors all do not know how to or desire to communicate events. Documented findings of failures and successful attempts to accomplish something avails teachings, for future students, amazed with inquisitive minds. Many of which will find they are not accepted by [the] *former failures,* of brainstorming inventions or goals, proved to be frivolous. There will continue to be a way to improve or detect what was believed to be a waste of one's precious time.

On a recurring basis health will continue to be a topic often spoke-of not only emphasizing dilemmas/cures new/old. Communication will permit *laws* to be improved upon, newly created and mandated, securing the future for patients. Increasing physicians and other professionals career choices, for they that commit to genuine patient wellness. For centuries of seniors and other patients in facilities for shelter and care were disabled, impoverished, neglected and unwanted babies; these individuals require the same dignity of care as the wealthy, insured, and those paying cash, to produce harmonious existence, for generations to follow. Many of which will live on fixed incomes, *Social Security,* and *Medicare;* others will live on *State Funds, Credit Cards, Bank Loans* and borrowed money they may not all be able to repay. A small group of seniors will sell their homes, stock, and/or live from the interest of investments. A minority will continue to **starve under a bridge** before *begging* for help.

Survivors of ordinary lifestyles, parents of adolescents that have chose to go to war and others raising children in single parent households will continue to struggle. When the last dollar is spent, those giving nothing will continue to suck the last breath from providers; that is a criminal offense itself.

Household hit in the 1960s through 1990s with high unemployment, sought public assistance. The stock market crash of the late 1920s to 1930s proved individuals with guts and brains succeed. World Wars I and II and cold wars thereafter, including the Vietnam War are repeats of historic events, alerting youths to prepare while able-bodied for a future filled with uncertainty. A dismal history of the population has turned thoughts around to where individuals now think more about personal needs, in the future than the present. Finances improve only through saving, and trust funds for adolescents; the world may just be a place worth living in, to see it after all!

As with anything of physical or psychological concern *food, beverage, socialization, sleep, exercise* and *solitude* create a well-balance. Knowing and utilizing sufficient quantities of *each, adds years,* to many lives. One other way to stay alive and well is to prevent harmful agents noted as toxins (i.e.: foods, people, pets, etc.) from rendering individual beliefs and rights, for no good.

Usually individuals do not go out to romp with for pleasures, *to avoid* an injury. Synthetic machines or equipment similar to the real thing, such as: *mountain or rock climbing, skiing machines, video games* and such have been best-sellers to mimicking actual fun. With such purchases a person can almost have the real pleasure sort of the sport or entertainment without fear of physical damage.

There is only a *Good-Outlook* if we think about tomorrow, and act on our instincts. The more we think the more we need to refer back to history's documented data. Predictions are done by astrologers, gypsies, crackpots, grandmas, historians, and just about anyone with a fun loving desire to entice the unsuspecting public into believing predictions are real.

My overall reason for writing the book was to voice an opinion and to inform people, they are entitled to *medical and surgical treatment*, no matter how much money they have. This book really does *not* pass judgment on all medical professional. Basically, this book is just to clear cobwebs from my brain, to enhance my thoughts of a dream world, *where,* individuals live happily ever after.

Observations of **Real Facilities**

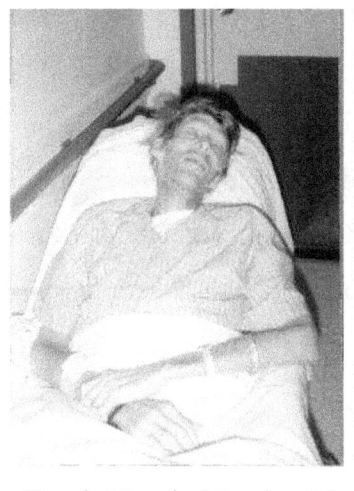 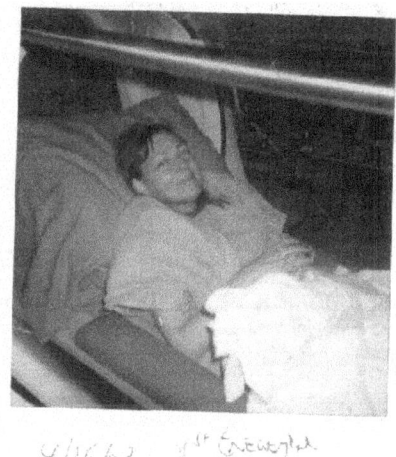

1999 My son Frank May in Nursing Home   2002 My sister 'hyperbaric' treatment

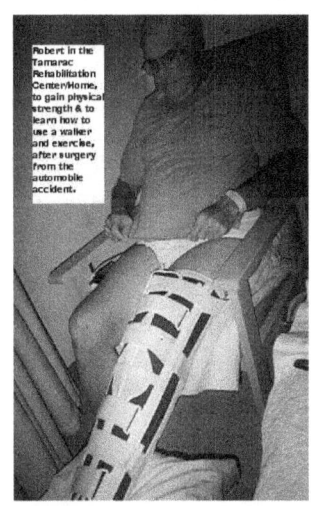 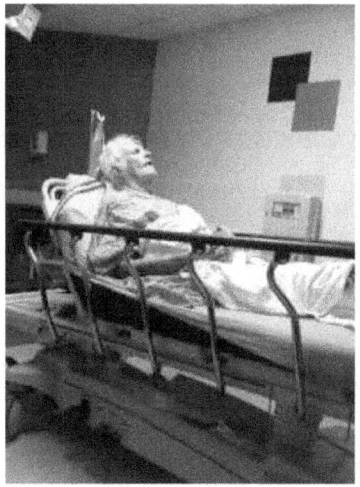 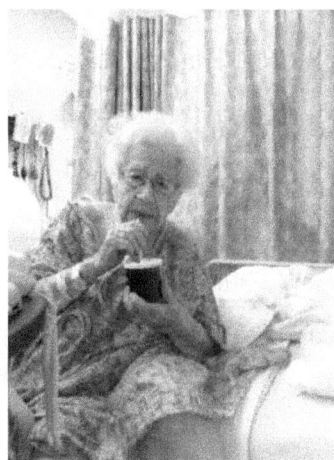

2003 My husband 2012 Pre 'TURPs'   2013 My friend

Yes there are numerous visits to others in medical facilities, each makes this book viable.

Although I did not work in *all* the places on the listed facilities; each for various reasons led me to observe the actions, during 1950s to 1990s. In my youth I obtained memories from medical/surgical treatment. I received, and as a volunteer I notice more. Other knowledge and observations have been acquired with related studies, during educational pursuits to improve my abilities as a caregiver. Comments on the list of places are clearly my own (personal choice); I probably should not include this section. Many of the facilities may have, to achieve better patient's concerns. Other may no longer be operating.

As a patient Some observations are negative. The way I feel patients should be *permitted* to be treated, depending on the abilities or levels of coherency differ from that of staff members (especially the graveyard shift: as in 11-12 pm till 7-8 am). Often with no insurance or minimal capacity to pay, for medical or surgical help, patients were and often still are treated with *a lack of concern;* similar to the way in which an unruly child is shunned by its angered parents, for a naughty or ornery action. Left to be self sufficient even though: unable or incapable of safely maintaining their self. My biggest complaint is the night shift, of many facilities while the sleeping staff hampers patient(s), from toilet use and leaving them helpless. During a crisis, patients are worse off than when at home all by themselves.

The data from research as well as personal observations and approximated dated-time (much by memory), does not in any way negate improvements that *may* or *may not have come to be* since. Some reference has been compiled by conversations overheard, by total strangers, as I individuals visiting friends or relatives; other orations were from those visited their friends or relatives, [patients]. Most of the data is *old-reference*; it has merit in-that when living becomes a threat, many have no way of knowing what to look for, in a permanent resting place (if unable to care for their personal daily needs). The places I have been to since the 1950s begins in alphabetic order, not, chronological. The list and throughout this book, I may have not clearly emphasized the staff often in morning hours were flooded with: '*student nurses* and *doctors*'. Students were working for credit hours, toward their degree, for clinical experience. They handled most of the patient care, studied patients charging opinions as analytical observations not excluding statements by whom they were assigned. Often they were writing reports which gave patients a negative prognosis, students not realizing some patients were not always aware of technicalities used to arrange tests or treatments, ordered by physicians, for whatever reason.

A Holly Patterson Home, Long Island, NY

A place elderly and disabled patients received long-term care. It had a beautiful garden area, dining and conference facilities for patients and staff, and it was equipped with at that time ultramodern technological mechanisms. Many patients require help to ambulate to the lavatory to bathe; other required assistance feeding themselves, have linens or clothing changed and laundered. A majority of patients were cared for by volunteers and assigned nursing/medical students, for clinically related studies (degree hours, class reports and research papers for passing a grade). I personally found *on-staff* members not happy with students, because it appeared patients received decent care, leaving the staff members as they were lacking. We [the student class in Geriatric Health Assistance] were certainly unwelcome. Patients requiring professionalism during treatments (i.e.: personal care), often were treated as if they didn't matter; they joked or just seemed to treat patients as inanimate objects. It was a horrible experience for the students [many discontinued the course]. It consisted of a crude and in-humane staff observing student practices, communications, and empathetic patient understandings.

I benefited by pushing aside awkwardness forming, to complete the course and received a certificate.

While studying and training for a Certificate in *Geriatric Health,* I observed this facility as being operated economically. Long-term [care] patients were each requiring assistance, for all daily living needs; a few were ambulatory. Most were bedridden. Equipment included: *weights, parallel bars, and diverse equipment* was available to patients rebuilding strength to arms and legs, for walking with crutches. There was a *hot wax treatment* and *aquatic therapy* department, to reduce stiffening joints of *arthritic* patients. *Amputees* confined to bed were given *body massage, therapeutic jet-spray spa baths, passive* resistant exercises, and many other treatments were available when sufficient staff and students were on-the-job. Attendants were more valuable than nursing aides [at times] because many patients were male, with muscular and heavy boned bodies. They needed two or three female aides to properly care for them.

There were elderly; weak and frail both genders in need of lifting from their beds, for personal care and to reduce stress (physically) from being in one position. For young, aides and attendants there were a few hoyer machines; also called hoists. This equipment (or machine) was a blessing during a single-handed patient care, for experience, in a 1 on 1 situation. However, the students did not receive assignments of heavy or clumsy patients, as a team of one, more than once. It was difficult but not impossible to position this hoist leveraging equipment, however, it reduced physical stress for student(s) and patients. Much of the therapy given was physical with a touch of psychological smarts when patients became depressed, disgusted to live with no arms, legs, and bodily functions, and many were just tired of being cared-for, as a infant (because of their physical condition).

Those patients diagnosed with Arthritis were taken to the therapeutic department several days a week; each student had to experience the wax treatment first, to understand why it was of importance to patients. And, believe me, it was the most soothing solution for my hands; the patients with large knuckles dipped their hands in the warm-to-hot melted wax. Not once, but a few times; allowing the wax solution to settle between dips. Once the wax on their hands dried, it was peeled away. The skin previously rough and dry was smooth and soft; stiffened knuckles moved with ease, not always 100% but with minimal if any discomfort. Although the treatments were required for some every other day, that was the one pleasure for many patients.

Electronic or mechanic beds were similar to many hospitals but for the patients with special needs, these were basic. Additional mechanical inventions were added to reduce the patient's need of full-care. The idea was to make living at this particular facility as near to home, as possible.

Studying [*for me*] *memo-writing, learning and incorporating ways,* to cope with the personal lifestyle (of oneself) with the task of seeing patients without limbs being kept alive brought deep-thoughts to me, and others. Students were told to interview patients during their scheduled assigned days. I found it to be one of the most difficult tasks; most patients with prosthetics were insulted, and felt their privacy was being invaded. Elderly confined would tell tales, often, imagined or embellished, to bring misery into a pleasant view, to students. Deciphering fact from fiction, well I guess that was secondary to the fact many confined folks were not wanted by their offspring. Some were deserted by loved ones not because of their old-age but contrary, family embarrassment often was the characterizations following those disfigurements, from an accident or incident, such as military injuries. Psychological and physical awareness was not an expectation of nursing students; many wished only to get-through the clinical care assignments and continue on with advanced studies.

Mentally incompetent patients carried conversations with or without anyone in their rooms, at times; some became violent, as students and professional staff members efforts failed to correct momentary disorientations. Prescriptions ordered by physicians reducing effects of long-term confinements, but for those with truly limited mental capacities, drugs quite often enhanced negative reactions. Violent patients were cared-for or treated with at least two aides; of which, one was always supposed to be a professional [on-staff].

The emotions expressed by some patients were hateful, to laws passed in Congress for pro-longed life as long as patients were *brain functioning*. However, there were not many patients with such skill or access to newspapers; those aware enough to view televised broadcasters/radio commentators knew they were unwanted. In 1975 it seemed cruel and inhumane, to maintain unwanted or debilitated individuals that had no desire to live, to me. To others, and to scientists, patients were the gateway into development for survival. Therefore, for me, writing good or bad observations with *opinionations*, it may seem improper to prolong life when there is little or no-hope of rejuvenation – to mind or restoration of body. Yet, it has been medically and surgically proven, some patients learn to deal with just about any negative aspect including amputations (of one or more limbs), deafness, muteness, and blindness. It has never been proved an adult male or female should have to be given false hope, for an indefinite time-span; somehow, "***keep a stiff upper-lip mate***" as the British say, can in deed reduce mental anguish, for both patient and caregiver.

Bellevue Hospital, in New York City, NY

A facility for the very poor. It was operated I believe by the city with municipal funding; I was too young to know or understand the politics of adult staff, yet, I visited a patient there and was disgusted & frightened. The place stymied my interests, therefore, this section is not updated or critiqued professionally nor researched or explored on the Internet. Anyway, during the 1960s and/or 1970s it was a stage for, moviemakers, and lunatics. I visited a friend with my mother – that was a patient there in the mid-1950s; that was an experience I'd rather not mention. But, for the sake of being fair, as follows: the facility/place was dirty and dingy with an odor that just didn't get any better than a city-dump. Individuals wearing uniforms, pastel blue (for students and aides), white starched dresses and hats (for licensed nurses), surgical greens (for operating room personnel), and jackets/lab coats (for doctors), was the norm as they promenaded throughout the building to their departments and stations. For me, knowing the uniforms came easy, from my stay in a hospital years before. Back then hospitals and similar medical or surgical facilities used similar uniforms, to identify the employees.

The beds were old, metal with hand cranks (to raise or lower knees/head). Guard-rails were metal, too; often used to tie patient hands or feet with restraining cloths, to prevent them roaming, removing tubes or scratching bandaged wounds. There were horrible green painted walls, striped halfway going around the building. There seemed to be a jail type of place, for those mentally insane individuals, with metal gate-like enclosures. It was a frightful thing for a kid to observe. It left lasting negative thoughts; thoughts, I hope never get viewed by others. Nurses Stations were filled with clutter (charts, telephone, intercom systems, a typewriter, and bulky switchboard room connections), for nurses to know about the patients. Smiling faces didn't seem to be available toward visitors, something I longed for, as a child (during a hospital stay years before). I thought it was a privilege to visit someone ill as well as a good deed. I thought it was a deed deserving a response, perhaps recognition a smile or pat on the back would have been sufficient. Even banks gave kids {*adolescents* not goats} a lollipop for showing up with their parents, back then!

Such recollections I have been keeping to myself, those miserable feelings of adults directed at adolescents (not only me). The nurses hated working there. I guess they had no other job to attend. The hospital was large, it took up what seemed to be a mile of walking distance, from the entrance to where the patient (we were visiting) was. There were old men in a *ward* (a room filled with numerous beds and patients). Each looked as though they were starving, frail and dirty (needing to be washed/bathed and shampooed, shaved, hair combed and clothes laundered). *Tube-feedings* were in some of the men's arms, and in nostrils of a few. *Foleys* dangled along the bed's metal frame filled with urine (smelly, cloudy, yellowish-orange urine). *Linens* soiled with either juice or blood or urine, as well. Not a pretty sight - nor site! Not a place I would send my parents [or anyone I felt a concern for]. I knew then and now, after years of seeing similar places, my feelings are the same, *there's no place good enough to treat most patients.*

[*independently*]

I am aware that I too cannot give perfect treatment or care, I admit that; but I know not to permit a person to be left unattended, for long periods of time when their capacity for survival is limited. Even the most difficult patients are only ornery with some people; with others, they are putty in their hands as those filled with clay, of a sculpture, by cosmic or karma, radiated professionally. Things I observe (that bothered me in my youth seemed to progress throughout my life while studying and working in various facilities. Some thoughts reverted to comparisons led to many voiced opinions, unacceptable to supervisors; frequently lacking staff because of municipal and private reduced funding. *Volunteers, students: nurses and doctors* were available; often opinions disregarded, by professionally exhausted staff and administrators. Its part of their position to create both a physical and mentally sound place, an atmosphere to encourage good health even under stressful conditions such as: *impoverishment, low wages, poorly equipped treatment rooms and areas, and patient over-load* – that is why staff and administrators receive salaries, to cope! Simple facts that I don't think cost too much are really a matter of striving to permit individuals to be human beings, not poor slobs – ***but just ordinary people.***

For example

– *clothing and personal grooming sometimes requires nudging*, patients that appear less than interested in their personal image, as viewed by peers. *Dietary requirements* everyone knows, nobody will die from only fruits and vegetables still somehow, I think a decent *meat meal* is important. *Beverages served* in facilities such as: iced water, fruit juices, milk, tea or coffee are good; every once in a while that iced cold beer is better than a zillion dollars, to some patients. *Friendly conversation* non-facility communications – to the most difficult and often unpleasant patient – are goods way to keep mental alertness active. Not only from other patients, the staff is trained to converse with patients for more than just clinical inquiries; conversations create data to treat the cause of emotional stress. Often stress and loneliness prevents patients from recuperating at satisfactory or anticipated time-span. Not all patients need psychiatric or psychological evaluations to understand poverty has hit them harder than a ton of bricks; however, staff and administrators have shed guilt for patients, of limited to nil – funds. {**That was then**}

Broward Community Medical Center, Broward County, FL

A lovely looking place, on the outside; there are plants, trees, two entrances. One has a ramp for wheelchair or gurney access. The other entrance is plush, in my opinion. There are glass doors [to entrance ways] leading visitor or patient, to a lobby not like other hospitals I had seen. The facility is equipped with not only patient minded treatment areas; it has a McDonald's Restaurant, a Banking ATM area, and two information desks. The lower level is designed for access to visitors, couriers, delivery people, and staff members.

Wheelchairs can be accessed if necessary for patients, first entering to be examined. The emergency room is open and equipped with many technologic mechanisms, equipment, and fairly modern personnel. Staffing is professionals guiding students, either residents or off-campus doctors, nurses, and technicians. The Radiology Department has several rooms for films and readings with doctor's offices being shared, during the viewing for diagnostic expertise. The equipment in offices throughout the building seems modern and quite often, updated. *Network computers, fax machines, telephone, etc.* are for the staff and personnel as well as students. The staff from what I have seen (only as a visitor briefly, and a courier assistant), have been friendly and primarily, sincerely genuine within their scheduled positions. The facility is a county funded hospital, means: ***funds***

are low but patients received quality care (even the poorest), were not detectably neglected.

The facility from what I have heard, in conversations between staff or visitors, is: '*a trauma designated medical center. In 1998 somebody fell on to the train track as a train passed; the person was injured, and brought to Broward County for trauma care.* Patients with no place to go, in need of medical care, for either physical or psychological purposes are permitted with assistance for an employee (or two) to have fresh air time. They get to walk outside the building and smoke a cigarette or two, and they observe the real world, as it passes on a recurring basis. It seems pretty nice, even thought being a patient isn't. There had been a clinic, which closed or moved to a new area in the summer of 1998; its demise eliminated individuals from hanging around the west entrance/exit area. [*1995 to 1998 both patients and curiosity observers had been permitting to merge in conversation and when necessary, use the facilities bathrooms, roam about the lobby and dine in the restaurant*]

Columbia-Presbyterian Medical Center, upper-New York City, NY

Wow, this place, I know everything and nothing at all about. It was a huge facility, in the 1950s and 1960s; students of medical and surgical studies during that time when I needed emergency care and reconstructive surgery, leaving memories to fill more than a few pages. It may still be there today as it was; it may have become equipped with modern technologies and other improvements. The way I remember it: there was several clinical area sharing the facility's campus. There were also hospitals and schools of studying within the building (campus). There were libraries for patients, students, and doctors. In the lower, underground level there was a pass-through-hallway type of dark area to lead residents and students to dormitories. In the basement there was also a big, beautiful chapel (or church) permitting staff, patients, and visitors {I assume – *within the community to attend religious services or silent prayer*} for blessings

156

on a weekly, regular basis. One Sunday morning, I was wheeled to the church, by an assigned, nurse. The place was jammed with people. My wheelchair allowed me to get up front, to see the service take place. The singing was great; everyone sang (except me), in tune to the hymnal and organ player. I couldn't yet read all the words, so I just sang what I remembered from listening to others, prior to my injury. It was a pretty nice place, considering, it was in a hospital setting.

The doctors, I shouldn't mention them because they were trying to be professional students, and this is just what they were – **student**. *Students* (third year residents) performed and trained students about the *physiological systemic activities*, of the human-body. I was just another of their guinea pigs (so I thought, at times). Documentation of pre-op and post-op changes (*improvements or decline in condition)* from the surgery {they had done, *to reconstruct my face and redevelop my hand*} was unmentionable. I felt intimated, insulted, and embarrassed by the scars, I couldn't figure why the wanted photographs. Now, I know, journalizing is an essential part of documenting growth and development as well as recuperative and rehabilitative procedures.

Several years ago, I decided to see what the hell those photographs showed. I didn't expect to even find any pictures *but* I found a picture of my scarred hand, in one of the medical books at the Library in Southeast Medical Center, in North Miami Beach, Dade County, Florida; the area was where I lived and worked as an aide, raising my children. One of the doctors and I spoke from time to time, and the conversation about my scarred face became focused upon. I was told the library was accessible to medical students and employees locally, so I mossied in a couple of afternoons, for a literary find. During 1996 and 1997 SEMC which was a Pharmaceutical Facility merged with Nova University, in Broward County (Florida). Much to my surprise, I doubt anyone would know the picture was of my scarred, young hand. I didn't look for other pictures on me (back then) because it is really an emotional thing. The reconstructive surgery consisted of skin grafts, from some areas of my thighs, hips, and low back. Transplants of hair follicles and possibly bulbous cell formations, were performed by suturing thin layers of skin with hair (and/or cell tissue) to the grafting site; my face or hand were also skin graft sites, to reduce injury's scarring. However, the surgical procedures were not perfectly completed. Numerous scarring presents me as a less than intelligent person; such frustrations have become the norm, for me. Rising educationally, casts much negative over-views to medical-surgical personnel (for both: *students and professions*).

Although I had been asleep during procedures, the pain was not felt physically; however, long and drawn out psychological years followed, to cope with being disfigured with some improvements. The recuperative time post-op was of course woozy, vomitus, and often very uncomfortable. Still it makes feel I was a lucky person. Not lucky to have needed skin grafts for reconstructive surgical procedures, but in an odd-way, that I was used as a guinea pig to improve techniques, for other burn and badly disfigured adolescents or adults. Enough about my experience (as a nurse's aide) because this book is not about me! Well, there were many other adolescents that had been treated for imperfections, to outgrow their miserable childhoods. A was clinic setup for outpatient care, once they were released from the Babies Hospital (division of: Columbia-Presbyterian Medical Center's campus).

The CPMC not only did surgery, clinical studies, religious involvements, and outpatient treatments; it also had a rehabilitation and educational facility on the upper-level. I had attended classroom like studies there, to learn how to write with my left hand (after surgery, to my right hand); all of this reeducation was done during my youth (while I was at an elementary level). I guess most of my teenage years were trying to figure out **how and why** I was scarred and precisely, for what reason was reconstruction unavailing itself. Unanswered questions I sought from within because I knew of my family had insufficient finances; led to such fear by relatives (that I had to learn to live and remember some lie [without the true facts] they wanted me to tell, to cover somebody's ass). And I don't mean it arrogantly, just fully, or anyway other than realistically true!

At one point while I was a patient there was a priest declaring me dead and issuing the last rites (or something). I was very much alive but with bandages covering my face, tubes in my arms (with blood, and other liquids), my hands tied to the bed rails, and heavily sedated there was nothing I could say or convey, to defer that incompetence. I heard my words in my head that I wanted to say and I thought I was speaking but yet, there was nothing being conveyed. That was a very frightening experience then (and now, as I think back, it still happens to be scary). I am alive. I have been alive forever and my oldest son was born in that same hospital. And, it was a delightful experience, to know, they didn't need me anymore for their guinea pig; I finally needed them to see how very alive, I was living with the scars, emotional trauma, questionable occurrences and other confusing contributing factors, that may never be clearly understood or acceptable (least of all to me, a person that saw and heard – all the crap there is or was); however, my future continues with numerous unexpected or anticipated success.

Experience

Yes, it's the best teacher; I have plenty of it. Other facilities below do not need to be commented about, least of all by me. They have and will always need patients, funding, and guinea pigs (human and animal); but individuals need to be treated with something more than inhumane care. Here goes another negative personal lived experience.

Coral Springs Medical Center, Broward County, FL

Some nurses aren't concerned with patients care, safety or anything, I have found as a patient here during the mid-1990s. The Emergency Room was great. The doctor had me feeling a little better after a breathing problem; my husband drove me to the facility for treatment because we had been visiting friends in the area. Once I was stabilized, admitted to the respiratory floor, and monitored via electrodes things were very different. The food was great if you like eating frozen stuff (that hasn't been seasoned or cooked properly). An assigned doctor did nothing; not even responded, to a phone call. Apparently the patient over-load was too demanding. When a doctor (assigned by the facility) did eventually return my call, several hours into the following day, the bothered attitude, in his voice gave me shivers. The doctor expected to be paid some astronomic fee; one hospital visit does not in anyway constitute payment of hundreds of dollars for a service not needed. He did nothing; no prescription was written, advised nothing in regard to speeding my recovery, and he sent me numerous bills. The rest of the staff professionally did project or convey their superior modern-world technological abilities, in a crisis. As my breathing increased with reduction for a need of respiratory therapy, slacking-off occurred. I wrote the miserable occurrence somewhere in the previous chapter, or the one before. My experience was personally a disaster. And, it did not stop there.

Personal observations from my bed of patients in nearby rooms calling for nurse, dinging of call bells, and howling yells of: "*help*" could be heard in far away lands; somehow the nurse's station did not seem to hear anything more than their staff's conversation about who was dating whom, and what they were going to do and how so and so met someone etc. I walked from my bed to the area, listened and spoke with a couple of nurses mentioning the patient in a nearby room was seemingly in much discomfort. It didn't expedite a rapid halt to the intense conversation. It was as though, that: "*...smiling thank you face*" was surgically imbedded, hmmm...!

Golden Glades <u>Convalescent Home,</u> North Miami Beach, FL

(formerly <u>Royal Palm Convalescent Home</u>) I was employed there for a year of so during 1979 to 1980; *blah*! Graduate nurses awaited - licensing from the State of Florida; they were not equipped to work in facilities, such as this. They wanted to be glamorous, get paid high salaries, and return to where they were born. Nursing Aides were in demand big time, nobody wanted to wipe away soiled buttocks or groins of incontinent patients.

Licensed and Graduate Nurses felt it was beneath their educational standards; aides and attendants were considered the low-lifers. Hmmm…! We were assigned the worst patients, day after day – shift after shift – double shifts when disgusted co-workers just gave up. Well, the pay was below minimum wage so the administration provided sandwiches for the graveyard (midnight to 8am shift) employees, and brunches for those remaining on double-shift status. When the paychecks were issued, frowns were cast upon those with more income than the owner. Oh, well!

Greynolds Park Manor Rehabilitation Center, North Miami Beach, FL

It was more or less a Catholic Home; not a terribly bad place, in physical observations. I worked there in the latter portion of the 1960s, and again during the latter part of 1978 to 1979 (part time as a second job). Patients were guinea pigs (experiments for *drug action, reaction, and interaction*). Emotionally disturbed patients were kept in a locked area called <u>*Section D*</u>; they were frequently sedated, to permit quiet for the nursing staff and aides taking care of them. ***Drug or alcohol dependent patients*** were treated with respect and care, according to the level of financial or political status and clout, they carried. Other patients especially the elderly (with average or complete working mentalities) were treated differently than those diagnosed psychologically impaired. Rehabilitation and Occupational Therapy gave them - the alert and aware of their surroundings a majority of the time – days of being creative, to continue their alertness. There were parties for patients and other social events but the nicest part about the facility; it was located on a piece of property over-looking a park with a lake. It looks like *Gracie Mansion or a place from the park's view for a Presidential vacation spot,* for fishing or solitude. This facility was a Catholic religious place without the weekly practices of the religion. The registered nurses were military-oriented, not only attire, physical gaits, verbalized communications, and harshness as they were indignantly assigned to a rat-hole. The more elevated professionally, the less compassion and understanding of the aides was projected. Working there could have been much more self-rewarding had the licensed personnel omitted their '*air of holier than thou attitudes.*'

Heritage House, North Miami Beach, FL not a place for: *patients* requiring good care. Here there were smiling receptionists but that was it. The director or whom ever employed staff was not willing to give me an interview or an appointment of any kind. Another negative aspect of Americans seeking employment and speaking only one language, in Dade County; ***Spanish*** is a prerequisite it seemed then, and not it has become the norm! That's annoying. With experience, education, and a working background in medical facility care of the elderly or disabled, I took the refusal to interview me as a personal insult!

Lincoln Hospital, Bronx, NY one more municipal or county hospital - in 1964, my mother moved to the area; I volunteered to work there (*as a nothing, just a volunteer to contribute my time in a small way for the care and treatment that I had received during my childhood and adolescence*), for a few weeks. I wanted to get the feel for the medical field, to see if I were cutout for the daily care of others, and possibly to pursue a career in helping others. It was at times frustrating. There were times I'd visit my mother and little sister and brother; the building they lived in was no nicer than that shabby hospital where I had volunteered to do menial tasks. The Bronx was a predominantly violent location. For my mother, her spouse, and two youngsters the building was the only non-Hispanics rental within their financial bracket (*low to nil*). Her neighbors were more courtesy minded than the patients, and the staff in the facility. My life back then should have been dissuaded from furthering a career in medical care facilities and these past few years of research and references combined in a book. However, it was an excellent and intimidating over-all experience. A was assigned to the Emergency Room, issued a pink smock, and a meal ticket to cover the first three day a week stint. My allocation of time was my choice, and it would have been longer had I not been a mother and wife (also). Not long after my first week, the place was robbed at gunpoint, by what seemed to be drug-addicts. I knew nothing about such types of individuals but learned there are many unacceptables that make others miserable.

Meadowbrook Convalescent/Nursing Home, North Miami, FL Still another, horrible place to keep the elderly hidden away from the outside miserable world; if that in fact is as terrible as being a patient for many confined till death. Many patients there were confined for medical recovery periods, and for them, then the moved on to their private dwellings – if they were fortunately enough to have owned anything. Others remained indefinitely, they have no-place to return and nobody wanted to be caring for them (as they progressed into older than thou ages). *There was a Meadowbrook Hospital or Medical Center in New York on Long Island; the name changed to Nassau County Medical Center – parallel to the count jail-house in East Meadow, Levittown, Westbury, a triad of cities utilizing the facility for advanced educational professionalism, family-care management, and the inmates also were able to be treated* – during an ailment. This enormous structure appears from the exterior view as being a high-rise but it is in fact a medical facility with dormitory and research laboratories, to join the community in advancements.

North Miami Convalescent Home, North Miami, FL It was within walking distance but the usual story, they were not taking applications when I went there seeking employment (near to where I lived, to save transportation costs weekly). I did observe the patients, at that time briefly. Many were in better physical condition than I had seen in the Heritage House, Golden Glades, and Greynolds Park Manor. The reason, it was **privately funded.** Minimal funding was from state and federal money.

Parkway General Hospital, North Miami Beach FL hmmm…! Employed there for almost a year, in the Radiology Department, I found non-patient care gratifying. It had no emotional concern, for the safety and well-being, of those requiring 24 hour observations and assistance. The hospital and pavilion did have patients and they were cared-for with humanitarianism. Patients brought to this facility as emergency patients or physician request (for: *testing or evaluations*) from Retirement Centers, Nursing Homes or Convalescent Homes (for suspected: *accidents or mistreatments*) soon recuperated. Many were returned from whence they came and were re-neglected, again and again, in a never-

163

ending, vicious cycle. Accident or private patients somehow felt the warmth and understanding that this facility radiated. It's now 1998 and the buildings have increased to handle the influx of patients. New additional departments have been added and the name has been changed (in the last few years). Currently, this facility is named Parkway Regional Medical Center. Indeed, it is a place to admire, and to rest assured your care and treatments will be nothing less than excellent.

Tamarac Convalescent/Nursing Home, Tamarac, FL I almost applied for a job, at this facility because I live nearby. It doesn't have that *oomph* I was looking for in a job. There seems to be an *air* of: "***don't intrude in our business***." That tells me there is no-good going one behind the closed-doors; and I found, it was impossible to snoop around. I tried. Believe me it's like Fort-Knox. It wouldn't be proper for me to hop the fence or sneak in a window, but I have been tempted. It is located just a few blocks north, of the City's Fire Rescue and City Hall buildings. Maybe I'll collect the real scoop on this place in the future, if I have the mental energy. For now, this book is nearing its finale'

University Medical Center, Tamarac, FL has been one place to be sick, and not feel as though as a patient, the staff is burdened by your presence. This place is wonderful. The emergency room personnel were great when I was gasping for air, with oxygen and an intravenous begun by the EMTs in 1994 or 1995; and were is only the beginning to the atmosphere there. The personnel may change; they are as eloquent as the _Parkway Regional Medical Center_. And, frankly, this place is better because I live down the street; there ain't anything better than convenience.

My experiences: *as a patient, mother of a patient, and a visitor have been nothing less than professionally encountered with the greatest humanitarianism*, for a local facility. Patients that require long-periods of-time waiting for test-results are not somehow left to feel trashed. The overall treatment collections and comparison in the book, from the 1950s to the 1990s conveys this facility is better than other facilities. Patients are treated and referred to physicians that use sliding financial scales for billing purposes; this reduces their financial burden out of pocket, but more importantly –

psychological stress is not increased when patients recover, from their ailment. Individuals in this hospital's area (dwelling-wise) are not as well off, as they pretend to project. Many elderly, on fixed incomes barely have sufficient funds to live from year to year. Medicare and Medicaid are the typical funding source, for the elderly as well as financially deficient households. Parents with adolescents often can afford School Accident Insurance but not much more; they are not treated differently from those with higher incomes or insurance through employee payroll deductions. The school [affiliated but not related to the school board types of] insurance pays a major portion with the balance if not paid by parents, absorbed by Medicaid or the hospital - **itself.** Someday maybe I will be able to make a monetary donation, for the care and treatment I have received here (it could be my contribution to the medical world for previous health costs I had not been able to pay). Something this facility and Parkway have in common, both have personnel and administrators that treat visitors with respect and do not get upset by a person's request for a cup of coffee (during a visit to a patient) especially during a crisis.

University of Miami/Jackson Memorial Hospital

Convalescent/Nursing Home Two facilities located in Miami FL I wish I could write things about but cannot. My experience in the UM/JMH facility was nearly as horrendous as ***Bellevue Hospital*** in New York. Patients in misery, in the hallway of floors designated for ***Maternity Care***. The smell of urine, fecal matter, soured milk (either from lactating mothers or dietary trays left stagnant), blood and mucous reeking within the air; I wondered how sanitary conditions had become denigrated. ***Emergency Room***

Corridors filled with patients moaning in pain, crying and not being attended, others ranting and raving with no professionals available to treat them. ***Ambulance and EMTs*** arriving with additional patients, as though a war had created a crisis; somehow, each newly transported patient was issued when a person was not busy a form to fill-in their name, address, reason for being in the emergency area; a rare patient was issued a gurney. There were none empty, from my observations. There was no way for anyone to allocate what was not in the building. Over-crowding by patients with or without parents and/or a consoling pal, developed into overwhelming chaos it seems; not once, but quite often. Each time I have visited a patient in the hospital it brought deep concern, and forced me to not write any specifics events. It was not my job. And, now, it is not my obligation other than morally and humanely, to convey the most odd-ball-ish observations in a book that also informs anyone reading this book in the future, that ***life certainly does – stink!*** The university has too many department and sport-affiliated divisions, with far too many individuals wishing to be professionals without practicing; this is not a good thing. However, the UofM/MJMH has gained global recognition throughout some the 20th century, not for patient care in a direct way. It was written up as the ***best surgical facility*** in the world. Heart transplants, kidney transplants, and such tediously surgical procedures have created a living façade to a municipal and county funded facility, incapable of dealing with numerous lesser requirements. Its affiliated long-term care facility, several blocks away also does not in any way (that I had viewed) project caring for those infirmed, unable to care for themselves. Many patients were placed in such facilities as indigents, welfare recipients, and with Medicaid funding there was no federal or state authority to complain to with any hope of – aide to those in need. Pretty sad when profession of medical facilitators turn there back on the local community's population in the 20th century, a time or era when the origination of community health had been around for 100 years and more. Yet, this place and as I have conveyed minimally, numerous municipalities have no funds nor regard for the sick, elderly, disabled, and certain not me or you or anyone else!

Yonkers Cardiac [Convalescent Home] Center, Yonkers, NY

I think it's obvious I am not a novice about medical facilities, only when it comes to writing a book. The reason I left Younkers Cardiac Center blank in the original book is because my father had been treated so long ago, for several weeks, and he was returned to good health after a severe heart attack. It was during late spring or early summer, of 1962. He was returned to almost perfect health, after his stay there. He came home only to die, after a month of so with a final crisis. As I remember from several visits to see him, there were old guys sheltered there; many had no place to live. They lived there and were content, nobody bothered them, and unfortunately, very few individuals seemed to know this place existed. For the good and decent treatment they gave my father, I am thankful. The more places men and/or women have with such emotional caring the more individuals will not need to have attorneys, to sue … for malpractice, neglect or other inhumane crap.

Up-dates as of April 2003

When my computer failed to be returned last week, from the repair center I decided to stop typing on the laptop and await my desktop's return. Going to the local library (resource center), the following periodicals re-affirmed, completing this book without waiting for the desktop to be returned. And I, much to my surprise, have a good (much more) gratifying researched data, to add. Nothing in regard to the facilities mentioned previously; however, data in the medical industry to improve conditions and patient care.

[4]***Business in Broward***: 2001 unveiled <u>Digital Mammography Units</u> at a cost of: *$921,000.00*; and a *four million dollar* bequest was a reflection with the Sister of Mercy, attending sees, as a patient; he was a philanthropist. Funds were welcomed, by a considerably large group of people. The beautifully designed and architecturally definitive work (of HCH's building structurally) reflects both religion and professionalism. However, beneath that façade, realism of the flaws of within personnel - is recognizable. The 587-bed, facility has since seen many changes, from its original opening to the community's patients in 1955, as the only Full-Service Catholic Hospital. Furthermore, since the religious – medical facility opened with a limited staff its growth has escalated to 600 physicians in 40 specialties. Hmmm…!

[5]***Business Week*** Spring 2003 there was no reference to volume, article number, or page other than … in the Outlook Section of the "**50**"

> … major-break-through by Medtronic Scientists found a solution for reduced scans and high-electrical shock *pacemaker patients.*
>
> The drug-eluting stints are (according to author: John Carey with Michael Arndt) healing devices by the activation process keeping the artery lumen, from reducing in size during a blockage, may develop into a stroke. {*this paragraph is not a direct quote by the authors; I rephrased the medical lingo for a better conveyance of the major importance to this finding*}.

My focus of the cardiac improvements does not negate the systems such as: pancreatic care - for *diabetics*, audiology – for *deaf*, nor ophthalmology for those with diminishing *visual-images;* my seemingly fixation with <u>cardiac and senior citizen care</u> stems from a lifetime of personal endeavor, to achieve open not only eyes and ears, but to personally observe major improvements.

It may appear pharmaceutical and technological manufacturers are more concerned than facilities filled with patients – when it comes to medical care. However, with Congress questioning new technological prescriptions and/or equipment - such can delay patients from receiving much needed adequate care. But, it does not single-out the patients doom that is the created failures, by over worked, under paid, and those employed in facilities to enhance or glamorous their personal images.

[6]*Kiplinger's* (Personal Finance), April 2003, vol. 57, no. 4, pg. 78, by Kimberly Lankford

Medicare v Medicap: Congress developed *MEDIGAP Plan* in ten variations. Regional Medicare costs fluctuated within the Northeast regions, having escalated costs second only to Texas, for medical care. The Southeast region remained more affordable with the Midwest close behind. However, Northwestern, Southwestern and particular regions were not included, in the article, specifically. Joining American Association of Retired Individuals [*AARP*] with or without prescriptions and medical memberships included, does grant 10% discounts, in numerous pharmacies, travel paths, and related member services enhance both physical and psychological impact for aging people. Furthermore, a local decrease in senior citizens encompassment on a regular basis, for medical insurance with AARP may become a problem in the future (for the company).

In addition to the above, my research has increased the dollar value of policies, of current day with may not be reliable in the future. Many patient dollars may continue to grow within purse-strings of the patients, assuming, ample insurance coverage is within their policies.

What with Medicare, and its tacked-on HMOs, contributions are very much taken-advantage of with each healthy year of their life. Statistics and Charts can be viewed displaying a much more in depth understanding by Weiss's report on the website: weissrating.com (according to the article).

[7]***Business Week***, April 7, 2003; pg 75-79

Would it not seem logical to return dietary-regimes, as preventive ailments, into patient cares? The lack of it (according to me) increases risks to young and old without discretion. This article states the lack of calcium from potatoes, which seems less than professional; as many students were that in science classes during the post elementary phase, educationally. However, has potassium was conveyed back then to be beneficial to humans, a decrease in nutrients has been noted, with the underground growth of potatoes omitting proper development of nourishment.

DNA: researched by *GENVAULT* retrieves samples of complete criteria and random samples, for research. The process known as: ***dynamic archive*** links with the aid of robotic equipment. The company is projecting, a law enforcement community for this technological forensic data reference – to convey leads in assorted legal reports and pertinent criteria.

[8]***US News***, April 7, 2003, vol. 134, no. 11, pg. 35-36 *Small Pox; Reduced Vaccinations to Dogs*

The article recommends cardiac patients, to steer clear of the vaccinations and immunized have suffered fatal effects; two females died, both were nurses. Each within a few days had fatal-heart attacks. The vaccination has proven to be hazardous and additional side-effects for military personnel at a 10 to 350,000 ratio developing inflammation in and around their hearts.

The government nixed vaccinations in other *high-risk* individuals with high blood pressure, elevated cholesterol, or diabetes.

Dog owners according to **Trend** claims annual *CORE* injections can be administered every three years instead of annually because it can cause severe adverse reactions, as well.

[9]*Architectural Design*, for the first quarterly edition in 2003 did not display disabled entries, often essential for patients recovered from ailments, such as: extremity replacement with prosthetic devices, use of wheelchairs and walkers at home, nor did I notice any improvements for elder-care. However, it is not a medically designing periodically, therefore it is not required to research and develop private dwelling conveniences.

The Future

The 20th century prepares its finale. 2000 will open the 21st century the onset to a higher-recognizable modern and technologically excelled atmosphere, with many more blank areas and locations to develop. Individuals have fears leading to mental anguish, by potential disturbances anticipated. They believe *"life isn't going to be good."* They believe money will be less valuable than desired and previously anticipated. **Truthfully**: *"nobody livers forever. Who'd want to?"* Nobody take money or possessions to the grave as done in ancient demonic ears. **Let's face facts**. *"There'll always be: **crumb-snatchers, rug-rats, and loved-ones needing help**. There also will always be a time when the wealthiest are worth less than the 'Lincoln' penny or the --- **we flush down the toilet.**"*

So *living or dying* {I preferring: **dieing -** *I probably typed incorrectly, its 00:07 – October 29, 1998 and I'm tired but at the end of the book - I may as well continue. It's probably dying or something stupid to confuse individuals with a fair mind*}. The two words, nothing more in common than a <u>value placed upon one's experiences</u>. This book is only one valued treasure I have kept to myself, to avoid seeming - incompetent. I have blurted out arrogantly, things from time-to-time that irked me. My observations are depressing (I admit). I have written simple facts (in this book). Other real-truths remain in my thoughts. For instance: ***I plan on living to be as ornery and happy as all other old and decrepit people, that I have come to admire, for their bravado-ism.*** I, myself laugh at me, my mistakes, and the mistakes others because I have come to realize the old-saying: "…**there're two sides to every story!**"

Glossary

References

Instructors, professors and other intelligent individuals [that] really need or love this section, look for: *their names, articles, and recognizable places.* This data is suitable, for conversation dinner parties. Often teachers read this section, to be sure students do research – or can verify data. Individuals even look because they have been trained to do so; to find plagiarism and report it, so somebody can be sued and money or some valuable asset crosses somebody's palm.

Some look to say, "*...they or we looked, and so on.*" An still many others look for a bibliography because they have been taught to write a correct term paper, often required to gain credit *where educational and professional credit is do.* Truthfully, if you are in this section – *of my book* – you are either a boring person like me or an important part, of this book.

I researched: *periodicals, newspapers,* and *encyclopedias; memories of years in and around medical facilities, has been included.* Some observations cannot be verified (unless a slue of individuals, rattle cobwebs of their minds which may create major hostilities). I don't think it's worth my effort to prove what I lived. I avoided certain emphasis in regard to some treatments were disgusting and abusive; if I included my youth treatments – I'd have a hell of a lawsuit and I'd become financially wealthy. Hmmm...! Yes, there are wealthy individuals with less than I; somehow, wealth can be compared to beauty – the person casting judgment has the only opinion that counts.

I say: "*Whatever, nothing can be done to remove half a century' experience and observation!*" Catch the list of references and rationalize the value of healthcare (both preventive and actual); knowledge can very well save hours and funds, from being eradicated.

The Random House College Dictionary, 1975 publication; New York, NY

Taber's Cyclopedic Medical Dictionary, 1975,12[th] ed, Davis, F.A.; Philadelphia, PA

Grolier's Encyclopedia [CD in BCC Library System]

Britannica Encyclopedia [CD in BCC Library System]

Compton's Encyclopedia [CD, personal computer reference]

[1] Hospitals & Health Networks, April 20, 1996v70n8p59(2)

[2] Medical Economics, Oct. 13, 1997v74n20p37(8)

[3] Journal of Nervous & Mental Disease, Aug. 1998,v1186p455-461(8)

[4] US Census Bureau's, Apr. 5, 2003,www.uscensus.com

[5] The Census Tract is the Census Bureau's, Apr. 5, 2003,www.uscensus.com

[6] Business in Broward, Jan. 2003, v17n1p27 [Health: Holy Cross Hospital]

[7] Business Week, Spring 2003 [Outlook Section of the 50]

[8] Kiplinger's, April 2003, v57n4p78; Kimberly Lankford [Personal Finance]

[9] Business Week, April 7, 2003; pg 75-79

[10] US News, April 7, 2003, v134n11p35-36

[11] Architectural Design, 2003 "1stq"ed

[12] personal years of experiences, research, and observations, 1950-1998; updates: 1999-2003 (as noted in 4 through 9 references)

U.S. Census Bureau (2015); http://www.census.gov/

Barter System, (2015); Yahoo$^{©}$Rakuten Loyalty,. www.Get.Smarter.com/barter system

Index

5:36:45 PM Tuesday, August 04, 2015

Today I have been home for a full 24 hours, from University Hospital. Friday July 31st 2015 I was admitted from the emergency room, after transportation, by EMTs. The purpose of my 911 call was numbness at waking from sleep, in morning time. The numbness did not disappear nor decrease for an hour. Contacting my primary physician in PMC (Plaza Medical Center) Sunrise FL, on what to do. Dr. Ruiz, primary physician advised to get a CT Scan; possibly, to diagnose a I was having a stroke.

- The hospital did in fact not seem to view a stroke; therefore, admission for observation, a neurological examination led to an MRI/A the next morning.

- I was very nervous and almost refused the MRI/A, as I get claustrophobic. The neurologist prescribed a sedative to calm me, and fear was overcame. That result did display 'a small stroke' so I am thankful I did not chicken-out.

- I continued remaining in hospital until Monday August 3rd 2015; I was discharged. A new prescription was added to the collection of medications already used, at home; this one to prevent clotting and additional stroke activity, of a lesser degree.

- Inhalers although a normal daily routine for pulmonary conditioning had not been puffed, since Friday morning; not even a rescue inhaler was used, by me. The hospital provided inhalation therapy two or three times a day, which decreased stress in my lungs. *Shortness-of-Breath* did not become a negative function till home, to which I did not as yet require inhalers, to breath easier. Rather I just sit and perform breathing exercises, to catch my breath.

Tomorrow I have scheduled primary physician's appointment to follow up the care required in the future. (Reddock, Lana 2015; include with most recently added data)

August 24, 2015 It seems rather generalized to announce that the in-hospital care during the time I had a stroke, was transported to University Medical Center's emergency room, there was no negative details to disclose.

As a matter of fact, no inhalers have been puffed on a regular-daily basis either. It appears the treatments, bed rest, and normal 'at home' activities have not stressed, pulmonary disease condition. At least for now, becoming Short of Breath is a tolerable concern daily; therefore, when I feel overly stressed the available inhalers (Dulera and ProAir) are used. But for the most weekly use, only once every few days is it necessary.

On a much more interesting and valuable medical care and treatment concern, my youngest son researched chiropractic treatments, in my area locally. And thus his research has not gone unused. I contacted the individual last week, an appointment was scheduled, and X-rays had been done on Friday, August 21st 2015. That office visit was pleasant enough; little stress psychologically surfaced.

After a weekend of pondering what should I expect about my spinal, results were better than I anticipated. The images (side view and posterior view) displayed not such a terribly out of place vertebrae. There is a little upper spinal deviation to the cervical thoracic area; there is also a little lumbar sacral vertebrae concern. This morning after the consultation the first chiropractic realignment procedure was performed by Dr. Armand Rossi.

Amazing that his communication verbally was absolutely correct, regarding the way I felt during the procedure. There was a slight dizziness when the procedure was completed, as the bed lifted electronically, to a standing position. Yes, it amazed me that the small office initial view from the outside was just a store front. Rather, this office has numerous rooms, for specific requirements.

- A front area for patients awaiting doctor's treatment, consultation, or scheduling a next appointment; not only chairs, an erasable white board with memos, a table filled with periodicals. Not at all done yet – there is a 'camel' seat that just makes for small talk conversation, during the waiting process.
- There is a doctor's office, for consultations with patients and caregivers.
- An X-ray room, which is equipped professionally, to minimize physical stress on patient's body, during the imaging process.

- The treatment room, a narrow but ample walk around area, permitted the patient to stand on a platform and hold onto hand grips, as the doctor lowered the bed. The equipment is amazing, filled with leather and electronic manipulation, which does not stress physically the doctor nor any patient.
- A refreshment room was shown to me on Friday, which provides patients coffee and whatever small snacks that might be nice during their waiting room time.
- In the hall area was a tall 'library' area, which had bookcase with several shelves filled. The books could be borrowed by anybody, and returned after reading.
- It almost makes little sense not to attend this office visit, just to say 'hello' as there is much to do.
- Furthermore, there is a 'kiddie korner' to entertain youngsters with a toy box of interesting stuff.

Needless to mention that this year, or perhaps this time in my life, so much improved attitudes and displays of "welcome patients; come on in" just overflowing with warmth. Of course this will be the place I have multiple vertebrae adjustment treatments, for the improvement to my dwindling spinal column's condition. And if I am fortunate, several months of treatments will become gradually decreased from several times a week, to eventually once weekly.

Although this gung-ho attitude of mine is gushing with a reverse, to that of previous experiences, in the medical field … perhaps, honesty does not always require negativity to suggest or clearly define good from bad care to patients and their medical professionals.

Today is September 14th 2015 and I am heading to the chiropractor's office shortly, for a treatment. In the afternoon a dental appointment for cleaning my teeth, and final a long walk for my dog Caj will require use of rescue inhaler puffing. Exertion from walking a block or more creates a shortness of breath that just does not ease up. But, my dog should have a long walk occasionally, as he is truly a blessing.

And furthermore, today this book is to be uploaded, to www.createspace.com to become self-published. As the book is 195 pages, proofreading and spell checking is essential – during this afternoon. And the rest is history….

Abuse and Treatment

…seems to have meandered between impossible (on a tight budget) to possible when financed with no limit. Decent, humane treatment, in long-term facilities of private homes, has faced a back seat decades. This topic, conveyed via mass communication, dragged the public's view and desire to live, beyond an age of self-sufficiency.

Ralph Nader

…wrote the truth in the 1970s. His articles and research were wonderful and informative. The public was bewildered at the on-set of his bluntness. Some individuals believe old-age to be a downfall. His charismatic writing informed the world of neglect, in places many individuals had not expected; in fact, they were expecting to be treated kindly and helpful, by the staff prepaid through personal or payroll contributions. Individuals knew he wrote from the heart, his gut-feelings. He brought controversial awareness, not only to the public in a generalized realization; his findings alarmed the media and networks, to seek improvements and to commit their reporters to direct *honesty* when researching medical care.

I for one have found Nader's articles to be needed, deserved, and the foreground to improved facility centers. He brought fear to both *young* and *old*, in the privacy of their living quarters; extending his message(s) orally, in conversations between his listeners in public places not excluding restrooms, where many individuals still hide away with a newspaper, filled with controversial data. He succeeded as a man with a message; envied by some.

Currently

…the elderly, handicapped (referred to as being disabled), and ordinary visit libraries, shopping centers, pharmacies and recreational areas; many smile. They are happy to be alive. He (Ralph Nader) brought individuals into a Safe Zone (physically and mentally), by introducing the world, to a point-of-view beyond the historic 1900s. Those in the thirties and forties were starting to regret ignorance about the medical and surgical profession, as their family structure was left often hanging not merely financially - hanging by the aftermath of procedural treatments that was debilitating loved-ones.

Psychological scarring

From moment-to-moment status lingered far into the future, for many families. There has been limitations with possibly no-way those types of damages can be reversed. Often incompetent healers, along with teams of strategists including technicians, for diagnostic and prognostic input were students. Filled with concern and modern believers educational facilities frequently are hindered, by less than adequate professors, by deficient technological mentalities. These are the individuals we each trust during a crisis - minor emergency when our child or grandparents incur an injury as well as major occurrences, of life-threatening ailments.

These scientific beings, studying to become suitable and professionals' of tomorrow often have no funds to advance; struggling, many look their desire - *to be perfect* - in an imperfect medical facility.

- Why?!? May be asked when millions of Medicare and taxes are drained from the payrolls of individuals through federal, state, city, town, and private fields of work?

- Why? And, again, ***why indeed*** might I and a handful of others still be asking that in conclusive and insulting question, of our government the collector and allocation of funds distributors, of our money!?!

I as an individual have minimal replies, for such an enormous statement. It is only possible to find results as a group, in each town, city, state, and country-region. Projecting progress into the world of economics, our personal contributed finances, for the unique purpose of prepaying, for *superior* not mediocre medical and surgical care. Yet, through my data processing skills I continue outwardly to be an author, I too am concerned *how* and *where* my life's direction will proceed.

It seems a bit grim, currently, as I develop this book from a previously written manuscript, researched with a neighbor's daughter (a teenager diagnoses as being a deficiency learner). Well oddball as the mildly-slow progressive but functioning mind of the girl is said to be, her skills *technologically* are quite good - if not better than mine. Her skills for research is creative and complete. That tells me, nobody is always diagnosed with complete accuracy, deserved.

"***MY THOUGHTS***" by Lana Reddock

Reading my autobiography, of course, I wrote it, depicts a history of might have become a downfall; I was injured at a very young age. Emergency treatment and diagnosis immediately concluded the injury was too great for any full-recover, and my mental abilities would be retarded {ha, ha, ha} for the rest of my life; this diagnosis was not because of mental damage but through related-psychological impact, by peers and strangers.

It took many years for ***me*** to accept *myself*, to pursue with full speed a head action; today I prevail the wonders I have discovered. Slowly, after many years of studying computer skills, technology accessories for enhancing a document and conveying personal findings to other professionals, I think I am a success.

Over four decades I have achieved from minimal household skills of the average mom, to become a baccalaureate in science. Getting there was difficult. Remembering answers for <u>quizzes,</u> <u>tests</u> and <u>finals</u> devastated me; a total blank filled my mind yet somehow, research and documentation in reports, 75 to 95 percentage of test grades throughout most courses, and an inner perseverance acquired from numerous setbacks, pulled me into a position of leadership. A leadership that I alone wanted, and thus far has not repaid the costs of my education; however, I anticipate in the future decade or two my life will not only become a financially minimized personal burden, and it shall become a comfortable and satisfying accomplishment.

"Beware of Wolves In Sheep's Clothing" this book depicts not only the:

> "*would you believe what I saw?*"

It has been during its editing process, revised editing, and most recently influenced data updates that I too no longer question any of the memories that I as a patient, a geriatric health assistant, nor an individual advancing, educationally, life is not what we make it. **Life is what others divvy.**

Additional inclusions have taken great time to consider, before improving upon a book written, for personal and psychological boosting. The previous paragraph for instance, depicts how I knew there was wrong on-going's in _medical facilities_, of yester-years; this book might create a '_food-for-thought_' image.

Hopefully, my input will be not merely read; I would like each person reading and comprehending its contents, to evaluate their care facilities. No, I do not expect a zillion letters or emails with negative or positive vastness nor condition improvements. My goal is for everyone within their regional-location, to be prepared, for their journey, into a care facility in their future. A permanently carefree and troublesome place is what many envision, if they think about the decades to come at all. [_Let me stop rambling_].

After many adults

Moms and dads found themselves struggling intellectually; they returned to colleges and universities, as mature students. Often they, <u>including myself</u>, found young innovators and entrepreneurs. Numerous mature students had not considered what the true-meaning of those innovators or entrepreneurs desired to represent, of their skill levels. I for one found myself feeling inferior when using computers, in a laboratory on campus. Everyone it seems was half my age, knew things that made me angry such as:

- How to turn one on or off [_computer that is_] properly?
- How to save documents, preventing great loss, of dedicated processing time.
- My biggest downfall early-on was Internet communication & research!

Hence, the degree programs; first degree in my maturing adult lifetime: **ASPIS** (Associate of Science in Private Investigative Services). It was followed after a year-off, to catch my views with a second degree BS/BA (Baccalaureate of Science in Business Administration). Now it sort-of makes sense; furthermore, forming any technological opinion that's not quite on my level of former knowledge, has greatly benefited.

For that level to advance higher, there's the degree for M of Ed (Master of Education in Instructional Technology); a program for me in the future – that came to be achieved in September of 2005, in the American InterContinental University in Weston Florida (FL).

Now, for verifiable evidence, as it's called, <u>articles, videos, and more exposed fraud,</u> in medical facilities and the public was infuriated. Ralph Nader wasn't one of those average reporters believing in *self-preservation.* He didn't intentionally frighten individuals by telling it like it is or was, in the 20th century. Nader skimmed the surface; opened mental doors forcing awareness, not only in private homes but medical facilities and scientific institutes globally. Compiled, combines, and continued research with staff and individually, he and a handful of reporters developed reports to knock our socks off. I merely portray my single-visions and research within the chapters ahead, to inform readers of how and where their **Medicare, Medicaid, Pay Roll Insurance deductions, and some <u>tax dollars</u> go**.

In the 1970s Nader's theme for living '*better*' shook the public into reversing their aging-process. His theme sort-of, in a realistic overview, bestowed a recuperative path for living, as well as the dying process, for which we all have to come to terms with – hopefully, later on in our lifetimes. Focusing on dreariness may be bleak; it is obviously the future whether we recognize it or not. Everyone has a choice, face reality or live in a bubble world of their own; by doing so, they *go along day-by-day in a state-of-shock when occasional ignorance backfires during a crisis.*

A policy of individuals with self-concern demanded better medical care & physical well-being to become the norm, in: *Health Centers, Spas, and other routine exercising facilities.* Individuals were rejuvenated by vigorous physical fitness teaming, in neighborhood centers and casual groups. Gad-zillions of fitness videos – created - by popular actors and actresses sold to the public at minimal costs. The fitness businesses boomed. Doctors and nursing personnel with antiquated or non-individuals minded thoughts subsided. Health became a craze in just about every nation. The revolution began as a warning and ended with self-commitment (of: *temporary regimes*). Self-involvement led individuals '*to stay fit*' and '*to avoid being overpowered*' by "**wolves *in sheep's clothing***" {hence the title}.

Although using *Ralph Nader* as a reference to begin this book, it is not an intentional tribute, to his work alone. There are researched articles from newspaper columnists, encyclopedia references, periodicals and personal observations in this book. The ***over-all-view*** of comparison between previous care and treatments in private and public facilities of medical abilities made changes. In current time and future expectations; I only touch the surface for a predication, of what the population has to look forward to.

As with any futuristic requirement, access to malfunctioning equipment in schools of technology will continue; forcing students to learn engineering, rather than healing. With reversal of studies: *maintenance workers, caregivers/caretakers, attorneys, accountants,* and *advisors increase occupationally; leading to a deficiency within the medical field.* This criteria depletes the need for good medical personnel, which is often degraded, by legal ***malpractice, professional jealously, and financial fraud***, *do in-part to restrictions by rules and regulation*s, once believed as the stairway to success.

My book may not be proper ***English*** in technique or etiquette; rather, it is written from the point of plain English, the way I converse. With experience and studies both in school, employed, and a periodic patient I believe my input is valuable. I have a more than average background when it comes to medical-sciences; my diverse medical-related mentality formed ***early in my life***. Toddler years throughout adolescence and well into my adult lifetime experience have never quite ended with any one medical need, being completely fulfilled. My desire to improve its branching out followed into adult life. As a parent, I found myself lacking educationally; I embraced studying. It was difficult. I studied, worked, struggled financially, and survived the dimmest moments of life; I still believe health is a required field for everyone, to study. Safety is only the prevention of harm. Serving individuals decently is why salaries are paid. I availed myself to aid a relative's family during their ***Cancerous*** crisis throughout the ailment's duration; nearly four years. Experiences, views, misjudgments, and hopes of a theoretically healthy population sometimes, seem unrealistic. Yet, I, and others strive for just that! A world where: '*safety and good health, leads the way.*'

My credentials in New York (NY) and Florida (FL) advanced, into changing careers from becoming a nurse to opposite probables.

- 1975 Certificate [Geriatric Health Assistant] Hempstead, NY
- 1992 Diploma [Computer Business Application] Miami, FL
- 1995 Certificate [a correspondence study of Wicca] New Bern, NC
- 1998 Associate Degree of Science; City College of Ft. Lauderdale, FL
- 2002 Baccalaureate Degree of Science; City College of Ft. Lauderdale, FL
- 2005 Master of Education American InterContinental University, Weston FL

The levels of education mean nothing, when in my life I cannot meet an agreement to my future. The studies brought me closer to becoming a self-preservationist, far more than any ranged of multiple learnings.

I see *myself* as a wise and curious <u>aging individual</u>, instead of just getting older and awaiting heaven or hell. I continue to pursue doing for others. As a volunteer in the City of Tamarac FL, and Fort Lauderdale FL with Impact Broward (RSVP) a couple of hundred hours annually since 2005 or 2006 began an era to be proud-of.

Writing experiences has not increased economics, in any way at all. This self-publishing has created a marginal expectation, to achieve in one year numerous books; not all about professional needs and action. Other books are filled with collectives, which have been scanned and stored on my computer, to publish as a lifetime's self worth.

www.ingramcontent.com/pod-product-compliance
Lightning Source LLC
Chambersburg PA
CBHW080638180526
45168CB00008B/3210